BIOELECTROMAGNETIC HEALING

A RATIONALE FOR ITS USE

Thomas F. Valone, Ph.D., P.E.

Send for FREE companion '**BEMs CD**' for this book!
It has an audio-narrated BEMs slideshow and much more.
Send email with 'BEMs CD' subject and mailing address to:
IRI@starpower.net

Integrity Research Institute

nonprofit 501(c)3 organization
Beltsville MD

100% of the proceeds from this book is to benefit IRI

for Jacqueline, the naturopath

Acknowledgements are given to Charles Polk, Fritz Popp, A.G. Obolensky, Chukuka Enwemeka, Ilonka Harezi, Jack Houck, Marco Bischof, Larry Azure, Ralph Suddath, Bruce Forrester, Gene Koonce, Science News, Longevity, New Scientist, Bioelectromagnetics Society, SOTA, DesignMed CRC, BBC, Smithsonian, and electrotherapy websites like www.futuretechtoday.com , www.toolsforwellness.com , www.wellnesstools.com and others for their pioneering efforts

Bioelectromagnetic Healing: A Rationale for Its Use

Thomas F. Valone

First Edition, July, 2003
Second Edition, August, 2003
Third Edition, October, 2003
Fourth Edition, February, 2004
Fifth Edition, June, 2004
Sixth Edition, September, 2005
Seventh Edition, June, 2006
Eighth Edition, May, 2007
Ninth Edition, November, 2008
Tenth Edition, October, 2011
Eleventh Edition, January, 2014
Twelfth Edition, May 2015

ISBN 978-0-9641070-5-2

Integrity Research Institute
5020 Sunnyside Ave., Ste. 209, Beltsville MD 20705
301-220-0440, 800-295-7674
www.IntegrityResearchInstitute.org
Author biography and vitae on website

CONTENTS

Revised PREFACE

This field started for me in 1987 with a bioelectromagnetics instrument design portfolio that eventually comprised AC and DC gaussmeters, geomagnetometers, electrostatic and ion current meters (still sold by IntegrityDesign.com), ELF spectrum analyzers, and a Dental Vapor Ionizer. I was privileged to exchange viewpoints with Dr. Robert O. Becker about the possibility of measuring a brain's magnetoencephalogram (MEG) with off-the-shelf high-gain amplifier chips and of course, the effect of the earth's Schumann resonance on brain waves.

A year later, I befriended the Russian medical doctor, May Bychkov, who had finally been allowed to emigrate to the US in 1987. He had authored 83 journal and secret publications from 1948-1973 in Russian mostly devoted to bioelectromagnetics. One of his secret patents in Russia was devoted to a "system for remote influence of brain potentials on animal and man by means of modulation of radiofrequency radiation." This expert in a field that seemed to be just emerging in the US told me that electromagnetic medicine was utilized in medical clinics throughout Russia. In fact, Dr. Bychkov said, for example, if a patient came in with an ear infection, an electromagnetic device was pointed toward the ear for a few minutes to eliminate the infection. He went on to convince me of the wide range of bioelectromagnetic instrumentation that his country had already developed and put to use in the medical field.

The work I did a few years later with ELF Labs and a few others gave me greater respect for such therapeutic applications of bioelectromagnetic high voltage devices. However, it was the many lectures from Dr. Bob Beck that really impressed me with what a physicist and engineer can contribute to this field. Bob was famous for recovering bioelectromagnetic treatment devices, as in one case, a high-priced Russian therapy instrument, and then making inexpensive consumer models for the general public. Some of his work on the Kaali patent is an example of his thoroughness.

It is obvious to most of those who study this field that it really comprises "the medicine of the future." The sad and deeply disturbing truth is that it has already been invented and presented to the medical profession over one hundred years ago, here in the US.

Natural healing has become a popular topic for book titles. However, a neglected source of healing found in nature is bioelectromagnetism, the topic of this book. **We are electromagnetic (EM) beings** with electrical gradients storing energy as much as chemical gradients do in the human body. The study of the biological effects of electromagnetic fields (EMFs) has only recently been called bioelectromagnetics (**BEMs**).[1] Yes, chronic exposure (8 hours/day) to electromagnetic fields (e.g., powerline magnetic fields over has sometimes been associated with potential for harm to the body. However, there are many BEM instruments and devices re-emerging in the 21st century, based on high voltage Tesla coils that bring beneficial health improvements to humans with short term (5-15 minute) exposure. The Tesla coil class of therapy devices constitute *pulsed electromagnetic fields* (PEMF) that deliver broadband, wide spectrum, nonthermal photons and electrons deep into biological tissue. Electromedicine or electromagnetic medicine are the terms applied to such developments in the ELF, LF, RF, IR, visible or UV band. With short term, non-contacting exposures of several minutes at a time, such high voltage **Tesla PEMF devices may represent the** *ideal, noninvasive therapy of the future*, accompanied by a surprising lack of harmful side effects. A biophysical rationale for the benefits of BEM healing a wide variety of illnesses including cancer, proposes a correlation between electron antioxidants as well as a restored transmembrane potential and the NaK transport across cell membranes with ATP-production and immune system enhancement. The century-long historical record of these devices is also traced, revealing highly questionable behavior from the medical and public health institutions toward such proven therapeutics. Key sections are noted with a ☺ symbol to indicate importance. Summaries of several BEM inventions are included but not an exhaustive nor comprehensive review. This book should not be construed as an attempt to prescribe or recommend treatment of any kind. It reviews an electromagnetic medical science that is almost inaccessible to the public otherwise. Patients should seek advice from a qualified medical practitioner at all times.

Thomas Valone
Washington DC

---

[1] Bioelectromagnetics Society (founded 1978), 2412 Cobblestone Way, Frederick MD 21702. www.bioelectromagnetics.org

Chapter 1. History of Electromagnetic Medicine

Historically, as far back as 1890, the American Electro-Therapeutic Association conducted annual conferences on the therapeutic use of electricity and electrical devices by physicians on ailing patients. Some involved current flow through the patient, while others were electrically powered devices. At first, only direct current (DC) devices were utilized in the medical doctor's office for relieving pain and vibrating female patients who were routinely diagnosed with "hysteria."

Nikola Tesla

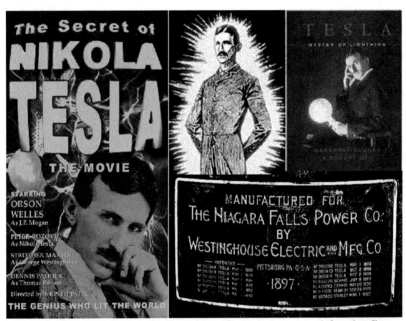

In 1895, the Niagara Falls Power Company opened for the first time and within a year, sent alternating current (AC) to Buffalo, NY (my hometown) twenty-five miles away, thanks to Nikola Tesla's AC generators. Cities throughout the world followed suit and made commercial AC power available to the general public, even miles from the power generating station. As a result, Tesla's high voltage coil devices, which were powered by AC, started to become widely known and applied.

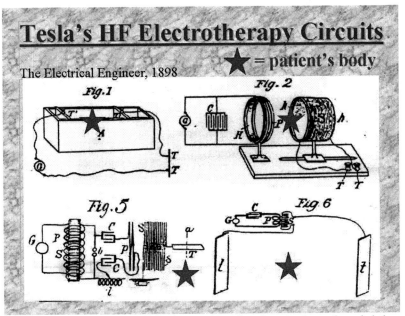

Tesla's HF Electrotherapy Circuits

The Electrical Engineer, 1898   ★ = patient's body

Fig. 1 *Fig. 2* *Fig. 5* *Fig. 6*

In 1898, Tesla published a paper that he read at the eighth annual meeting of the American Electro-Therapeutic Association in Buffalo, NY entitled, "High Frequency Oscillators for Electro-Therapeutic and Other Purposes."[2] He states that "One of the early observed and remarkable features of the high frequency currents, and one which was chiefly of interest to the physician, was their apparent harmlessness which made it possible to pass relatively great amounts of electrical energy through the body of a person without causing pain or serious discomfort." Coils up to three feet in diameter were used for magnetically treating the body without contact, though ten to a hundred thousand volts were present "between the first and last turn." Preferably, Tesla describes using spheres of brass covered with two inches of insulating wax for contacting the patient, while unpleasant shocks were prevented. Tesla concludes correctly that bodily **"tissues are condensers"** (capacitors) in the 1898 paper.[3] Today, the average capacitance of

---

[2] Tesla, Nikola. "High Frequency Oscillators for Electro-Therapeutic and Other Purposes," *The Electrical Engineer,* Vol. XXVI, No. 550, Nov. 17, 1898, p.477

[3] Condensers or capacitors are the terms for charge-storage devices usually modeled as two parallel plates that may have a dielectric insulator inside.

bodily tissue is confirmed to be about 100 – 300 pF.[4] It is also the basic component (including a dielectric) for an equivalent circuit only recently developed for the human body.[5]

The relative permittivity (an electrical property) for tissue at any frequency from ELF (10 Hz-100 Hz) through RF (10 kHz–100 MHz) exceeds most commercially available dielectrics on the market.[6] *This unique property of the human body indicates an inherent adaptation and an innate biocompatibility to the presence of high voltage electric fields.* It can be traced to the high transmembrane potential[7] (TMP) already present in cellular tissue. Tesla also indicates that the after-effect from his coil treatment "was certainly beneficial" but that an hour exposure was too strong to be used frequently. This has been found to be still true today with most of the Tesla coil therapy devices.

A year before, in 1897, Dr. Frederick F. Strong added a Geissler vacuum-tube containing rarefied gas to the high voltage output.[8]

In 1916, Dr. Sinclair Tousey published a large medical electricity textbook which identified only two forms of high-frequency devices used in medicine: 1) Tesla or Oudin high voltage resonator and 2) D'Arsonval high current design.[9]

On September 6, 1932, at a seminar presented by the American Congress of Physical Therapy, held in New York, Dr. Gustave Kolischer announced: **"Tesla's high-frequency electrical currents are bringing about highly beneficial results in dealing with cancer, surpassing anything that could be accomplished with ordinary surgery."[10]**

---

[4]   Sheppard, A.R. and M. Eisenbud. *Biological Effects of Electric and Magnetic Fields of Extremely Low Frequency*, New York University Press, New York, 1977, Ch. 5, p. 4-18

[5]   Polk, C., & E. Postow, *Handbook of Biological Effects of Electromagnetic Fields*, CRC Press, 1986, p. 58

[6] Fink, D.D., "Dielectric Constant and Loss Factor for Several Dielectrics," *Electrical Engineer's Handbook*, 1975, p. 6-36

[7] See Appendix for the details of the transmembrane potential.

[8] Strong, F. *High-Frequency Currents*, Rebman Publishers, NY, 1908, p.15

[9] Tousey, S. Medical Electricity and Rontgen Rays, with a Practical Chapter on Phototherapy, W.B. Saunders, 1916 (The best four chapters, totaling 250 pages of the book, is available <u>on CD</u> under the title, "Medical Electricity" from Integrity Research Institute - IRI #416)

[10] Obolensky, A.G. "Early Cancer Cures were Based on Mitogenic Radiation" Natural Energy Institute, 2001, p. 1 (reprint in Appendix)

Georges Lakhovsky

In 1925, Georges Lakhovsky published a paper with the explicit title of "Curing Cancer with Ultra Radio Frequencies" in *Radio News*.[11] His expressed philosophy was that "the amplitude of cell oscillations must reach a certain value, in order that the organism be strong enough to repulse the destructive vibrations from certain microbes." He goes on to say, "The remedy in my opinion, is not to kill the microbes in contact with the healthy cells but to reinforce the oscillations of the cell either directly by reinforcing the radio activity of the blood or in producing on the cells a direct action by means of the proper rays." Lakhovsky's Radio-Cellulo-Oscillator (RCO) produced low frequency ELF all the way through gigahertz radiowaves with lots of "extremely short harmonics."[12] He favored such a wide bandwidth device so that, **"The cells with very weak vibrations, when placed in the field of multiple vibrations, finds its own frequency and starts again to oscillate normally through the phenomenon of resonance."** As a result, Lakhovsky's RCO is now more often called MWO (multiple wave oscillator) for these

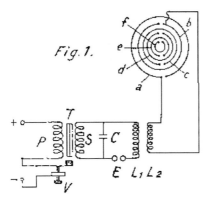

Fig. 1.

Figure 1
Circuit diagram from US patent #1,962,565 by G. Lakhovsky

reasons. The MWO uses a Tesla coil and special antenna with concentric rings with increased spacing that induce multiple sparks between them (Fig. 1) as seen in his US patent #1,962,565. Compact, portable, screw-in-lightbulb-style vacuum-tube upgrades

---

[11] Lakhovsky, Georges. "Curing Cancer with Ultra Radio Frequencies," *Radio News*, February, 1925, p. 1282-1283 (reprint in Appendix)
[12] Grotz, Toby, and B. Hillstead. "Frequency Analysis of the Lakhovsky Multiple Wave Oscillator from 20 Hz to 20 GHz," *Proceedings of the US Psychotronics Association*, Portland, OR, July, 1983 (see Appendix)

are found in his later US patent #2,351,055. Lakhovsky's article and patents are on line.[13] His book, *The Secret of Life* was first published in English in 1939. In 1949, a review of Lakhovsky's work was published as *Waves That Heal* by Mark Clement. Besides this technical information, the life of Lakhovsky is a study in suppression and summarized below in a paper by Chris Bird:

> The first man I will mention today is the Russian-born Frenchman, Georges Lakhovsky. I learned only yesterday that Lakhovsky seems to have been an associate, or knew, Nikola Tesla.... Georges Lakhovsky began to experiment with what he called a "multiwave oscillator." (In the Library of Congress there are some ten books written by Lakhovsky, all in French.)
>
> This multiwave oscillator (MWO) put out a very broad spectrum of electromagnetic frequencies. The theory, as propounded by Lakhovsky, was that each cell in the body of an organism—be it a plant, an animal, or a human being is in itself a little radio receiver and work on its own special little frequency. Each cell, in addition to being tissue, in addition to being biology, is also electricity. On that theory, he held that pathology was not a matter of biological concern or intervention, but one of electrical concern and intervention. He theorized that from the bath of electrical frequencies put out by the multiwave oscillator, each cell individually could and would select that frequency which it most needed to restore its equilibrium.
>
> So he began to experiment not with animals or human beings, but with geraniums. These were geraniums which had cancers—plants get cancers too. And, lo and behold, the geraniums were cured of their cancers; which simply began to fall off since they are external in the case of geraniums. The geraniums would just shed the diseased tissues when exposed to the MWO. Lakhovsky then went on to do work on animals and human beings and his work was picked up by

---

[13] Lakhovsky patents and February, 1925 paper online at: http://www.rexresearch.com/lakhov/lakhusps.htm (see Appendix)

doctors in six or seven countries, among them Italy, Sweden and Brazil. Finally, because he was on the "wanted" list of the Nazis, he was smuggled out of France and came to New York during the war, where he worked with a urologist. The record of his treatment of degenerative disease, with what amounts to an early "energy-medicine" device, was remarkable. But the work had to be done in secret because orthodox medicine did not favor this device, and its power, associated with that of the FDA and the AMA and other "control organizations," kept the MWO underground.

The Lakhovsky device is a very effective one. I'm not going to say that it's 100% effective because I don't think any device is, but it is way up there. Georges Lakhovsky died in 1944 or 1945.[14]

Today, Lakhovsky machines are commonly used in Europe. IRI has responded by becoming a manufacturer of a Lakhovsky Multi-Wave Oscillator with the Premier 2000.[15] The concentric MWO antenna can also be used in pairs with the patient in between them. In addition, a Neon or Argon gas tube applicator can be substituted or added to the antenna.

At a recent conference, I met a car accident victim who gave a detailed account of his visit to a therapist in Europe who gave him one treatment with a Lakhovsky MWO that lasted about an hour. He credits this experience with the subsequent lack of scars on his face. From a BEMs point of view, an explanation for the MWO effect on scar tissue might be the electron antioxidants which quench free radicals but mostly, the effect can be attributed to **the boost in TMP which are known to help Schwann cells create new tissue without scarring.**[16]

This author subscribes to the "**Lakhovsky Philosophy**" which bathes the body with a broadband of Tesla coil frequencies in the kHz, MHz, GHz ranges and allows the body to absorb the frequencies that it needs. It is different than the Rife Philosophy.

---

[14] Bird, Christopher. "The Politics Of Science: A Background On Energy Medicine," *Energetic Processes: Interaction Between Matter, Energy & Consciousness, Volume I*, Xlibris Press, Philadelphia, 2001, p. 226

[15] www.BioEnergyDevice.org, also see www.zephyrtechnology.com

[16] Becker, R.O. *Ann NY Acad Sci*, 1974, V. 238, p. 451

Royal Raymond Rife

In 1934, the University of Southern California appointed a Special Medical Research Committee to study 16 terminal cancer patients from Pasadena County Hospital that would be treated with mitogenic impulse-wave technology, developed by Royal Raymond Rife. After four months the Medical Research Committee reported that all 16 of the formerly-terminal patients appeared cured.

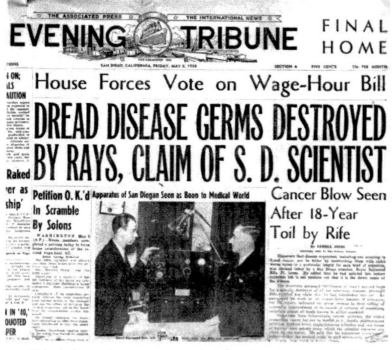

This information was concealed for decades by the AMA as pharmaceutical economics collaborated with the 1910 *Flexner Report* which literally cut funding for universities involved in alternative "medical" or health subjects. The *Flexner Report* boasting "analytic reasoning" still restricts pharmaceutically-based doctors today to a knowledge base conveniently limited to drugs designed to create dependency while electrotherapy alternatives that strengthen the immune system are available without the chemical "side effects" that presently plague modern medicine.

Rife's high voltage gas tube device was designed, with the aid of his unique microscope, by experimentally witnessing the effects on microbes and bacteria, finding what he believed were the particular frequencies that resonated with their destruction. "In 1938, Rife made his most public announcement. In a two-part article written by Newall Jones of the *San Diego Evening Tribune* (May 6 & 11), Rife said, 'We do not wish at this time to claim that we have "cured" cancer, or any other disease, for that matter. But we can say that these waves, or this ray, as the frequencies might be called, have been shown to possess the power of devitalizing disease organisms, of "killing" them, when tuned to an exact wave length, or frequency, for each organism. This applies to the organisms both in their free state and, with certain exceptions, when they are in living tissues.'"[17]

"He had the backing in his day - this was in the 1930's - of such eminent people as Kendall, a professor of pathology at Northwestern University and Millbank Johnson, M.D., who was on his board, along with many other medical men, when he began to treat people with this new 'ray emitter.'... There were articles written on the Rife technique... in the *Journal for the Medical Society of California* and other medical journals. Suddenly, Rife came under the glassy eye of Morris Fishbein of the AMA and things began to happen very quickly. Rife was put on trial for having invented a 'phony' medical cure. The trial lasted a long time."[18]

In 1953, Rife published his cancer report in book form, *History of the Development of a Successful Treatment for Cancer and Other Virus, Bacteria and Fungi*.[19] A turning point occurred in 1958, when the State of California Public Health Department conducted a hearing which ordered the testing of Rife's Frequency Instrument. The Palo Alto Detection Lab, the Kalbfeld Lab, the UCLA Medical Lab, and the San Diego Testing Lab all participated in the evaluation procedure. "All reported that it was safe to use. Nevertheless, the AMA Board, under Dr. Malcolm Merrill, the

[17] Lynes, Barry. *The Cancer Cure That Worked: Fifty Years of Suppression*, Marcus Books, Queensville, Ontario, 1987, p. 103
[18] Bird, p. 227
[19] Rife, Royal Raymond. *History of the Development of a Successful Treatment for Cancer and Other Virus, Bacteria and Fungi*. Rife Virus Microscope Institute, San Diego, CA, 1953 (see also www.rife.org)

Director of Public Health, declared it *unsafe* and banned it from the market."[20]

In 1954, John F. Crane, owner of the Rife technology, contacted the National Cancer Institute (NCI) concerning the Rife therapeutic instruments. Barry Lynes writes, "The Committee on Cancer Diagnosis and Therapy of the National Research Council 'evaluated' the Rife discovery. They concluded it couldn't work. No effort was made to contact Rife, Gruner, Couche, or others who had witnessed actual cures (Couche was still curing cancer patients at that time.) No physical inspection of the instruments was attempted. Electronic healing was thus bureaucratically determined to be impossible. In 1972, NCI Director Dr. Carl G. Baker used the superficial 1954 evaluation to dismiss Rife's work when asked for information by Congressman Bob Wilson of San Diego."[21]

In 1961, after a trial with an AMA doctor as the foreman of the jury, John F. Crane, the new owner of the Rife Virus Microscope Institute, spent three years in jail, ostensibly for using the Frequency Instrument on people, though no specific criminal intent had been proven. In 1965, he attempted to obtain approval from the California Board of Public Health for use of the Frequency Instrument. "On November 17, 1965, the Department of Public Health replied that Crane had not shown that the device was safe or 'effective in use.'"[22]

From 1968 to 1983, Dr. Livingston-Wheeler treated approximately 10,000 patients with the Rife Frequency Instrument, at her University of Southern California clinic, with an 80% success rate.[23] In 1972, Dr. Livingston-Wheeler published *Cancer: A New Breakthrough* in which she "condemned the National Cancer Institute for its misuse of money [$500 million in 13 years], the corrupt handling of public health responsibilities, and its use of people [100,000 cancer patients] as guinea pigs for a 'surgery-radiation-chemotherapy' program dictated by special interests."[24] Her last book on *The Conquest of Cancer* was published in 1984 in

---

[20] Lynes, p.129
[21] Haley, Daniel. *Politics in Healing.* Potomac Valley Press, Washington DC, 2002, p. 114
[22] Ibid., p. 133
[23] Ibid., p. 116
[24] Ibid., p. 117

which she celebrates the European acceptance of the Rife discoveries but complains about the situation in the U.S.

All of these distinguished scientists, back in 1958, had been carrying on significant research in the biological and immunological treatment of cancer for years. It is still only now that the United States orthodoxy is beginning to catch up. Because of the suppressive actions of the American Cancer Society, the American Medical Association, and the Food and Drug Administration, our people have not had the advantage of the European research.

This work has been ignored because certain powerful individuals backed by large monetary grants can become the dictators of research and suppress all work that does not promote their interests or that may present a threat to their prestige.[25]

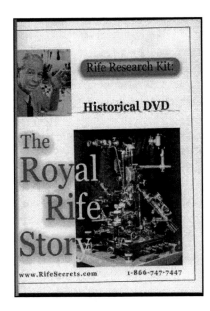

Rife died in 1971, mostly of a broken heart. For further details, one of the best historical documentaries of his life, including audio and video clips from Rife himself, is "The Royal Rife Story" on DVD.

Today, Rife machines abound in many varieties so that it is hard to tell which of them follow the original design parameters of Royal R. Rife. An early Rife technique of **using ultraviolet-killing frequencies, unique to each microbe** (also requiring eye protection during use), is taught in Dr. James

---

[25] Livingston-Wheeler, Virginia, and E. G. Addeo, *The Conquest of Cancer*, Franklin Watts, 1984

Bare's patent which shows the energy of UV for each microbe.[26]

However, Lynn Kenny, CEO of **Beam Ray LLC**, bought all of the Rife archive material from John Crane years ago and claims to have followed Rife's original work. The **Beam Ray Light and Sound Generators**, both desktop and portable, use computer-controlled pulsed infrared (IR) gas tubes. These EM terahertz signals have been proven to penetrate the entire body with little attenuation *even twenty feet away*. Such Rife technology, currently undergoing FDA approval, affects a wide range of conditions involving pain relief and pain management. It does not operate in the ultraviolet (UV) range which is a lower frequency than IR.

A portable product in the Rife market, using only pulsed red, blue and IR light is Lightoolz International.[27] Dozens of LEDs are mounted on a pad, like the handheld LightPodZ™ pictured to the right and pulsed at clinically tested Nogier frequencies such as 146 Hz, 587 Hz, 2349 Hz and 4698 Hz. A less expensive version (at 10% of the price) which I like,

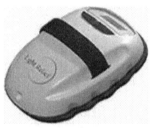

with very similar design and marketed for over ten years to sports doctors and professionals is **Light Relief** Model LR150.[28] It has AC-power or rechargeable batteries and selectable pulse rates of low, medium and high. The rubber LED base is detachable for easy placement under clothing while sitting, reclining, or while in bed and can be used for extended periods. It also comes with a built-in 15-minute timer.

Light Emitting Diodes (LEDs), which have become even brighter and more powerful today than ever, have been shown to bring relief to young cancer patients using a 3-by-5-inch portable LED array held against the skin and improve a bone marrow transplant patient's quality of life, with a 48% pain reduction, according to the Medical College of Wisconsin.[29] The LED array was made by Quantum Devices of Barneveld, Wisconsin, which has also been shown to aid in wound healing. Powerful LEDs

---

[26] See Patent #5,908,441 "Resonant Frequency Therapy Device" 1999

[27] See www.lightoolz.com and www.lightwandz.net for more information

[28] See www.lightrelief.com POB 3252, Hollywood CA 90078

[29] See www.nasa.gov/vision/earth/technologies/led_treatment.html

developed by NASA have been shown to heal wounds in lab animals and spur plant life in space. The FDA has approved a multi-year investigation of the LEDs as an experimental treatment led by **Dr. Harry Whelan**, Professor of Neurology, Pediatrics and Hyperbaric Medicine at the Medical College of Wisconsin. So far, he has found that diabetic skin ulcers and other wounds heal faster with the LEDs, which also grow human muscle and skin cells five times faster than normal. He states, "**The near-infrared light emitted by these LEDs seems to be perfect for increasing energy inside cells...and accelerate healing.**" Near-infrared light has been shown to penetrate the body to a depth of 23 cm or more than nine inches without damaging the skin. Though the LED that Dr. Whelan uses, developed by **Quantum Devices**, is three times brighter than the sun, the red light it emits, at three different wavelengths, is cool to the touch. **LEDs are known to stimulate cytochromes in the body that increase energy metabolism of the cells.** Cytochromes are part of the "electron transport chain" (see Krebs Cycle in the Appendix) that converts sugar into instant energy required by the body to perform all of its actions, such as raising a finger or healing a wound.[30] Even the Navy and DARPA have contracted with Whelan to start testing the wound-healing LED device.

More information on this topic of light and the stimulation of biophotons can be found in Chapter 2. It is worth mentioning here that all of the Wisconsin studies with LEDs simply used <u>continuous light</u>. Light is a form of energy that behaves like a wave with electric and magnetic oscillations (an electromagnetic wave). The development of monochromatic light sources (e.g. lasers) with single or narrow spectra of wavelengths continue to pave the way for more studies showing what doses and wavelengths are therapeutic. Evidence indicates that cells absorb photons (particles or packets of EM light waves) and transform their energy into **adenosine triphosphate (ATP)**, the form of energy that cells utilize (and a product of the Krebs Cycle).

Much discussion in the rest of this book indicates that pulsed and continuous LED light (e.g., 630 nm), as well as laser light, can have rapid and dynamic effect on cellular repair and healing.

---

[30] See http://tinyurl.com/q3yr6un - Dr. Whelan also uses LEDs to activate light-sensitive, cancer-killing drugs for treating brain tumors, without harming healthy cells.

Antoine Priore

Antoine Priore's electromagnetic therapy machine was perfected during the 1960's and early 70's as a team of leading French scientists demonstrated "conclusive, total remissions of terminal tumors and infectious diseases in hundreds of laboratory animals...funded by the French Government. The approach employed very complicated mixing of multiple EM signals in a rotating plasma, and modulating the mixed output upon a very strong rippling magnetic field to which the body of the test animal was exposed. Complete remission of the treated diseases was obtained. In addition, the animals' immune systems were also restored to normal...In the mid-70's Priore's work was suppressed, because of hostility of the oncology community, change of the French Government, loss of further funding, and complete inability of the physicists and biological scientists to even hypothesize a mechanism for the curative results."[31] This last reason reminds me of the book by Thomas Kuhn, who argues that a radical phenomenon in science will be repeatedly treated as an anomaly until a new theory can explain it.[32] Here is an insight into his life:

> I will tell you about one more person—still another self-taught genius, Antoine Priore, who began working in 1944-45, right after the war, to develop an electromagnetic device which cured cancer. He got the backing of some very interesting and courageous people, including the world-famous immunologist Dr. Raymond Pautrizel, of the Univ. of Bordeaux II, who did all of the animal work. When Dr. Pautrizel arrived on the scene, because the emotional atmosphere surrounding the cancer cure was so great, he decided to take the research in another direction and began to use the machine to treat what he knew best, which was sleeping

---

[31] Bearden, TE, "Vacuum Engines and Priore's Methodology: The True Science of Energy-Medicine" *Explore More*, Number 10, 1995, p. 16
[32] Kuhn, Thomas, (1970) *The Structure of Scientific Revolutions*, University of Chicago Press, 1970, p. 78

sickness in animals. Sleeping sickness was of primary concern to Dr. Pautrizel because it is a widespread affliction in tropical countries and, perhaps because he was born and raised in Guadeloupe in the Carribbean, he had become very interested in tropical medicine. When he injected rabbits with the pathogen trypansome, which causes sleeping sickness, the trypanosome would multiply until there were billions of them circulating in the bloodstream and the rabbits would uniformly all die within 72 hours. But, when exposed to the radiation of the Priore device, these same rabbits would live. Yet their blood was still teeming with the trypanosomes, which could be extracted from the radiated rabbits and injected into other control rabbits, which would then die.

This implies that the machine was doing something electromagnetically to the immune system of the rabbits such that they were able to fight off a lethal disease which would normally kill them in 72 hours!

Had it not been for the courage of Dr. Robert Courrier, who at that time was Perpetual Secretary of the Academy of Sciences of France, in the face of great criticism, the scientific data on 20 years of that work might never have been published. Time after time, over 20 years or more, Dr. Courrier personally introduced the papers for publication in the *Comptes Rendues* (Proceedings) of the French Academy of Sciences. There are 28 such papers. Even this could not prevent Dr. Pautrizel from nearly being fired from his post at the University of Bordeaux II, where he finally treated human patients successfully with the Priore device.

When he wrote a paper and sent it this time to the Academy of Medicine, it was refused without explanation. Pautrizel then wrote a long letter, since made public, to the governing offices of the French Academy of Medicine to find out why the paper had been refused and which people on the jury refused it, so that he could consult with them in order to better inform them of the facts. For 3 1/2 years he received no reply.

So then he decided to step outside of normal scientific channels and offered his story to a journalist who wrote an extraordinary book called *The Dossier Priore, A Second Affaire Pasteur?* Because the book has not been translated from French, and may not be (because it was written for a French audience and should really be rewritten in English) it is not accessible to English readers. But I have written a 50-page paper which is a synopsis.

We have discussed the cases of four intrepid researchers. Of these, three had no formal academic training—Priore, Naessens and Rife—and yet they went on to develop the most extraordinary medical tools in energy medicine that I think exist. Two of them were put to trial! One was nearly fired from his position. All this is moving and largely unknown medical history and all of it affords real opportunities for further exciting research. [33]

Robert Becker

A pioneering medical doctor in the 1960's, Dr. Bob Becker is most famous for his book, *The Body Electric*, which gives an autobiographical account of his life's experiences with bioelectromagnetics. [34] Not only did he establish that the Chinese meridians of the body are skin pathways of decreased electrical resistance but he discovered a host of other bioelectric effects within the body as well, such as electrostimulating limb-regeneration in mammals. He also worked on electrically stimulating bone growth with Dr. Andrew Bassett, who along with Dr. Arthur Pilla, developed a *very effective PEMF generator* to stimulate bone fracture healing, approved by the FDA with an 80% success rate.

---

[33] Bird, p. 235
[34] Becker, Robert O. *The Body Electric, Electromagnetism and the Foundation of Life*, William Morrow & Co., New York, 1985

Since bone is piezoelectric, these specially designed signals effectively create stresses that open the calcium channels, in the same way that <u>weight-bearing exercise does</u>.[35] Similar PEMF signals (see Appendix) recently have been used effectively to treat **osteoporosis** even in patients with an ovariectomy.[36] These three doctors inspired the OsteoPad™ that can now be installed under one's mattress to send **bone-strengthening signals** all night to bones and joints, in their own home (see Glen Gordon section).

Abraham Liboff

A modern-day physicist and inventor, Dr. Abraham Liboff is the discoverer of electric-field and geomagnetic ion cyclotron resonance, which more reliably explains the resonant interaction of static magnetic fields with endogenous AC electric fields in biological systems.[37,38] A physicist with Oakland University, he has introduced significant physics principles into the field of bioelectromagnetics. His "Method and Apparatus for the Treatment of Cancer" (US Patent #5,211,622) tunes an alternating magnetic field, superimposed on a static magnetic field, to maintain a combined effect that has the proper cyclotron resonance frequency so that the neoplastic tissue containing a preselected ion can be treated to bring about a decrease in the proliferation rate of the cancer cells. It also can be combined with a chemotherapeutic agent for a synergistic effect. However, it is noted in the patent disclosure that "up to 100 days of treatment will provide beneficial results."

☺ Glen Gordon

Dr. Gordon, a medical doctor, used to speak of the first critical 12 hours as a "stunning" situation in which a person's body is

---

[35] Bassett, C. Andrew, "Biologic Significance of Piezoelectricity", *Calc. Tiss. Res.,* 1, 252-272, 1968

[36] Chang, K. and W.H. Chang. "Pulsed electromagnetic fields prevent osteoporosis in an ovariectomized female rat model: A prostaglandin E_2-associated process" *Bioelectromagnetics*, V. 24, Issue 3, 2003, p. 189

[37] Liboff, A.R. "Electric-field Ion Cyclotron Resonance" *Bioelectromagnetics*, V. 18, Issue 1, P. 85

[38] Liboff, A.R. "Geomagnetic Cyclotron Resonance in Living Cells" *Journal of Biological Physics*, V. 13, 1985

responding to an injury. During that time, the body has to call upon what he calls a "constitutive response" – based on what is present – whereas after that first 12 hours, the body has had time to produce additional elements, called the "transcriptive response," being transcribed from the DNA and produced into building blocks of regeneration and healing.

Thus, the most crucial time in which the PEMF technology can make the most difference – even life and death, is in the first 12 hours in which the PEMF can help the body manage the overwhelming release of **free radicals** as a result of the stunning trauma which causes **inflammation** that is connected to cell damage. He also addressed in his lectures on DVD (e.g., "Speaking of Your Injury," the stress from a physiological perspective, citing that the mitochondria produce free radicals a stress situation.[39]

Gordon emphasizes that pulsed EM fields stimulate neurons to grow faster, citing a "watershed report" by NASA.[40] In 2003, NASA scientists found nanosecond pulses 2.5 to 4.0 times better than older pulse shapes at restoring tissue after trauma. This is due, among other factors, to nanosecond PEMF's marked ability to **stimulate growth hormone** and the Heat Shock Protein (**HSP70**) within 10 minutes, which is restorative and regenerative. PEMFs also supply natural electron antioxidants to neutralize free radicals rapidly. Free radicals have a role in aging, illness, and death. *Stopping free radicals stops inflammation.* "Healing won't take place until inflammation stops," he says. Dr. Gordon cites several scientific papers from medical journals that have documented that the EM pulses accelerate healing by acting as a catalyst to correct the alignment, making it easier for the antioxidants to connect with the free radicals.[41]

---

[39] Excerpted from Sterling Allan, "Glen Gordon Speaks on PEMF Developments," ExtraOrdinary Technology Confer., Salt Lake City, 2004, http://www.pureenergysystems.com/events/conferences/2004/teslatech_SL C/GlenGordon/ElectroMagneticHealing.htm

[40] Four-year Collaborative Study on the Efficacy of Electromagnetic Fields to Stimulate Growth and Repair in Mammalian Tissues, NASA/TP-2003-212054, http://ston.jsc.nasa.gov/collections/TRS/_techrep/TP-2003-212054.pdf

[41] Chang CW et al., "Tardy effect of neurogenic muscular atrophy by magnetic stimulation" *Am J. Phys Med Rehabil*, 1994 Jul-Aug; 73(4), 275

In 1980, his team received the first investigational device exemption issued in the US to study low-level laser effects in soft tissue injuries. After his staff scientists convinced them that the light was not penetrating the tissue, he had to admit that the accompanying pulsed EM field was responsible for the results they observed in rapid healing of injured patients. This led to the development of a hand-held battery-operated device called the "EMpulse," invented by Dr. Gordon, with an 8 nanosecond rise time, the fastest in the industry.[42]

His FDA-approved **EMpulse demonstrated a 40% increase in growth hormone**. He said the pulsed magnetic field penetrates the skin at least 4-5 cm but that there are other phenomena at work because he was seeing effects clinically much deeper than that. He subsequently treated over 20,000 patients using this technology. Dr. Gordon cited a Stanford study that showed **"onboard antioxidants were 100 times more effective."** It can treat inflammation, illness, and aging symptoms with no side effects.

The most dramatic demonstration of the EMpulse healing potential was the intervention in Gordon's own coronary disease in 2003. After retirement, he had several heart attacks, angiograms, and surgeries that still left him with severe heart pain whenever he exercised. In 2003, his colleagues told him that this doctor needed a transplant or he would be gone when the next heart attack occurred. Instead, he scavenged the Internet and found a medical article reporting the PEMF energy stimulated new blood vessel growth in heart muscle.[43]

Then, based on this information, he started using the EMpulse device by putting it in his pocket next to his heart for several hours each day. He was able to walk further and further as time went on and, as a result, never had the transplant. He experienced such dramatic heart function improvement that within six months, the elderly Dr. Gordon completed a **2,500-mile solo bicycle trip** across the country to show the world that he was healed. He appeared on several radio and TV programs along the way. Yet, cardiologists routinely dismiss his "anecdotal experience" and were unwilling to

---

[42] Gordon, Glen, "Designed Electromagnetic Pulsed Therapy: Clinical Applications", *J. Cellular Physiol.* 212, 579-582, 2007

[43] Yen-Patton GP et al., "Endothelial cell response to pulsed electromagnetic fields: stimulation of growth rate and angiogenesis in vitro" *J Cell Physiol.*, 1988 Jan; 134(1), p.37-46

discuss it. It is also unfortunate that a bioelectromagnetism course is not included in medical students' curricula, so doctors in the 21st century do not have models to understand PEMF-tissue interaction. IRI has responded by improving his old EMpulse design with a larger coil and rechargeable battery in the new **EM Pulser.**

Dr. Gordon stated his frustration with the politics of the American Medical Association and the U.S. Drug Lobby who have stonewalled this technology from achieving acceptance by the mainstream of U.S. medicine. For example, he said that until Abraham Flexner's publication of "Medical Education in America" in 1910, consumer support for electromagnetism treatment was excellent, and Maxwell's prior insights in the 1860s had stimulated even greater interest here and abroad. But Flexner's "exposé" forced closure of 170 "proprietary" institutions with "irregular teachings" that included electromagnetism and other promising modalities. Mainly about establishing his own power, Flexner's coup ignored the science and *eradicated electromagnetism from US medical curricula.* This was accomplished despite the acceptance of Maxwell's electromagnetism work and its widespread use throughout Europe and the Soviet Union. The long-term effect from this historical shift in medical evolution is that today, are 2.5 million deaths a year from hospital-administered drugs, 200,000 of those are from gastric bleeding according to Gordon.

Dr. Gordon believed that electromagnetic pulse technology may eventually nearly eliminate the need for the pharmacological industry with intervention and prevention. In his Spring, 2005 newsletter *Explorer*, support for this ambitious projection includes,

> Dr Gabi Nindl of Indiana University School of Medicine praised PEMF's "potential to revolutionize medicine" at a Denver symposium on Biomedical Sciences in 2004. A solo study of genetically identical mice saw increased life expectancy of 15% (661 vs. 586 days) in the treated group.
>
> Dr. Deborah Ciombor, a scientist with fifty prior articles, noted in the June 2003 issue of *Osteoarthritis Cartilage* that PEMF "appears to be disease modifying in this model," chosen for its multiple similarities to human arthritis. Imagine, joint destruction stopped. Anti-inflammatory drugs and

arthroscopic "clean-outs" stop nothing en route to joint replacement, while the former alone kill 30,000 annually from bleeding.[44]

This technology has the potential to revolutionize medicine, according to Gordon. He also worked on an EMpad design, which was intended for osteoporosis patients. It should have been introduced to the market thirty years ago when Drs. Pilla, Bassett and Becker pioneered FDA approval for bone healing magnetic pulse devices and admitted they could be used for reversing osteoporosis. Integrity Research Institute has now completed an **OsteoPad**™ product to fulfill Dr. Gordon's dream and help the 50% of all elderly people who develop some degree of osteoporosis.

For health practitioners, Dr. Gordon cited a 1997 federal law enacted by Congress that allows "off label" use of a technology permissible (including PEMF devices) when done in conjunction with a licensed provider. After Dr. Gordon's passing and the end of the EMpulse production, this author re-engineered his device with a bigger coil but maintaining his famous "**nanosecond Risetime.**" The improved **EM Pulser**™ comes with a rechargeable battery, faster pulse rate, stronger signal, and a 30-day money-back guarantee. Both the EM Pulser and the OsteoPad are now sold through the nonprofit IRI website at www.BioenergyDevice.org and www.OsteoPad.org .

☺ Norman Shealy

A medical doctor who worked with Nobel Prize winner, Dr. John C. Eccles, Norman Shealy, M.D., Ph.D. has a journal publishing history extending back to his first papers in 1957 and neurophysiology papers with Eccles in the 1960's. He is the inventor of the transcutaneous electrical nerve stimulation (TENS) device in 1967, as well as the recent Shealy RelaxMate II. He is also noted for BEMS procedures that include Dorsal Column Stimulation (the control of pain by electrically stimulating the dorsal column of the spinal cord), and Facet Rhizotomy (the permanent, safe numbing of an irritating spinal joint nerve).

---

[44] Gordon, Glen. *Explorer*, Vol. 1, No. 3, Spring, 2005, p. 3 (several short videos of Dr. Gordon are available online at www.YouTube.com)

However, the most impressive achievement for longevity, that he discussed at a recent USPA conference where I was in attendance, is his Five Sacred Rings.[45] These are different energetic circuits associated with acupuncture points that specifically optimize DHEA, Neurotensin, Beta-Endorphin, Aldosterone and markedly reduce Free Radicals. The one that stimulates the *youth hormone*, DHEA, is called the Ring of Fire and involves a 50 gigahertz (50 billion Hz) signal device (GigaTENS or SheLiTENS) that touches the skin, two points at a time, at several points in the circuit. Through repeated laboratory testing for careful monitoring of DHEA levels, with the only testing lab in the country that varies less than 10% in its results, Dr. Shealy was able to confirm the protocol that **restores youthful levels of the master hormone DHEA** by stimulating the pituitary gland to produce it. Upon completion of this work, he theorized that average life should be 140 years of age. More recently he has demonstrated regrowth of telomeres, the tail of DNA. Telomeres ordinarily shrink 1% each year after birth. His work with the RejuvaMatrix™ (a high voltage Tesla coil device with a pad one can lay on top of) is the first to demonstration rejuvenation of telomeres, a major key to anti-aging and longevity.

His recent book, *Life Beyond 100: Secrets of the Fountain of Youth*, contains the details of this amazing life-extension BEMS discovery.[46] He also has a holistic university that offers degrees related to integrative health care.[47] Dr. Shealy is also organizing the

---

[45] DVDs of Dr. Norm Shealy's health secrets are available at www.normshealy.com .

[46] Shealy, C. Norman (1996). *The reality of EEG and neurochemical responses to photostimulation - Part 1 and 2*. Light Years Ahead: The Illustrated Guide to Full Spectrum and Colored Light in Mindbody Healing. Celestial Arts Press: Berkeley, CA. Edited by Brian Breiling;

Shealy, C. Norman (1996). *DHEA The Youth and Health Hormone*. Keats Publishing, Inc.: New Canaan, CT;

Shealy, C. Norman. (2005). *Life Beyond 100: Secrets of the Fountain of Youth*. Jeremy Tarcher/Penguin, New York ;

Shealy, C. Norman (Editor in Chief). (1998). *The Illustrated Encyclopedia of Healing Remedies*. Element Books, Inc.: Boston, MA. Element Books: Australia

[47] Holos University Graduate Seminary www.hugs-edu.org - See also http://www.normshealy.net/

first accredited Energy Medicine program in the country, available through Greenwich University and the U of Missouri.

Bart Flick

Probably the only protégé of Robert Becker, M.D., Bart Flick, M.D. became a co-inventor on a patent with him. At an electrotherapy seminar at Penn State University, he described some of the early work he did in wound healing. He said that the wound normally exhibits a positive voltage potential. Instead, he found that if a *-40 mV potential can be restored in a wound area*, which normally exists on the skin, **the healing rate is *twice as fast***. Since silver and silver colloid are known to have antibacterial properties, he said it was the perfect metal to put across a wound, *connecting it to the negative skin voltage potentials on either side of the wound*. The weaving of silver thread into nylon provided the best fabric to accomplish this task. Benefits are that Silverlon® cloth bandages (1) re-establishes a -40 mV potential to the wound by electrical conduction, (2) are a local antibiotic, and (3) exhibit a "tissue penetration effect" in glove and shirt designs. Related to the TMP, the skin potential is just as important as this invention shows.

For severe wounds and burns, a blend of nylon fiber and silver coated nylon fiber demonstrated advantages that are safe, convenient and long lasting, including faster healing time and extended use. While this author attending his lecture, Dr. Flick showed graphic photos at Penn State University of a woman whose forehead was severely lacerated after going through a windshield. He explained that scarring would be normal in this situation but the photos after Silverlon® was used on her were very impressive. A unique infusion of silver throughout a comfortable, flexible fabric delivers pure ionic silver to the wound site longer than other silver-impregnated products on the market. "Studies of the kinetics of ion release suggest that silver nylon may be an effective, sustained release antibacterial agent."[48]

Electrically generated silver ions have been shown previously to be a potent antibacterial agent with an exceptionally broad spectrum

---

[48] MacKeen, P.C., Person, S., Warner, S.C., Snipes, W., and Stevens, S.E., "Silver-coated nylon fiber as an antibacterial agent," *Antimicrob. Agents Chemother.*, 31, 93, 1987.

as indicated by in vitro testing. The MacKeen study reports on clinical experience using **electrically generated silver ions from Silverlon® fabric** as adjunctive treatment in the management of chronic osteomyelitis.

In tests conducted by a multi-site home health agency, Silverlon® was found to heal wounds rapidly, and decrease nursing visits and costs. "In one case, a diabetic patient in renal failure with a sacral wound, was showing no improvement after 20 skilled nursing visits. The physician was planning surgery. After a trial using Silverlon®, the wound healed completely in three nursing visits.[49] Dr. Flick also showed examples of bone infections that were healed with Silverlon fabric which do not respond to any other treatment, including oral antibiotics.

In medical jargon, "the combination of NPT and elemental silver contact dressings represents an exciting new method of securing STSG's in colonized wounds. Patient education and compliance in this more sophisticated method are issues to be addressed."[50] However, doctor education and compliance are even more difficult issues according Flick, who indicated that emergency room protocol is slow to change, even when it is proven that Silverlon® bandages provides superior end results and faster healing.[51] It should also be mentioned that for the same reasons, **silver colloid** nose spray and dropper bottle, such as the **Silver Biotics** product available through www.BioEnergyDevice.org, provides home therapy for killing viruses, bacteria and mold spores on contact by *electrocuting the surface of the pathogen.* We have found that **Silver Biotics** liquid is highly active form of the colloid since the average size is regulated to 10 microns. Fill an old nose spray squeeze bottle or dropper bottle with the liquid and prevent colds all winter before the germs grow in the sinus passages. One can feel it working on contact.

---

[49] "Treatment of Orthopedic Infections with Electrically Generated Silver Ions." *J. Bone Jt. Surgery.*, 60-A, 871, 1978, Becker, R.O. and Spadaro, J.A

[50] Sigler T, Patterson GK, Loehne HB, Sawyer A, Johnson P, Farmer M, "The Use of Negative Pressure Therapy and Elemental Silver Contact Layer in Increasing the Survivability of Split-Thickness Skin Grafts," Presented at the *16th Annual Clinical Symposium on Advances in Skin and Wound Care*, September 20-23, 2001.

[51] More information as well as the wonderful silver bandages are available at http://www.silverlon.com/

William Pawluk

An international authority on the clinical use of PEMFs which enhance acupuncture, homeopathy, low-level lasers, and other bioenergetic modalities, William Pawluk, MD offers a **Pulsed Electromagnetic Fields Workshop** to educate the workshop on this expanding and exciting field. He is also the author of *Magnetic Therapy in Eastern Europe, A Review of 30 Years of Research*, in which he states, "Three decades of work in magnetics, which has gone beyond the theoretical, suggests that there is indeed merit for their use – not only in their effectiveness, but also in their safety."[52] His early work with Drs. Bassett and Pilla involved pulsed electromagnetic fields applied to bone non-unions that were resistant to surgical intervention.[53]

Ed Skilling

A pioneer researcher and inventor in electro medicine, I have known Ed since the 1980's. In the 1990's, I briefly worked on the final touches of his handheld electric wrinkle reducer for ELF Labs, Inc. His life's work has been dedicated to healing the human body. From a very young age, Ed Skilling had always shown an exceptional aptitude for working with electricity. At the age of ten in 1928 Detroit, he constructed his first radio and has been building and experimenting with electronic equipment ever since.

Through an early experiment, he realized there were benefits to sound frequencies. On the family lawn, he transmitted radio signals underground from one copper pipe to another. To his surprise, the grass between the two copper pipes grew profusely. When he sent radio frequencies through soil planted with alfalfa seeds, he found they grew higher and faster than usual as well.

Ed trained as an electrical engineer, though his passion for engineering drew him to the fields of mechanical and hydraulic engineering. Rather than work in a conventional industry, Ed Skilling devoted his efforts to his true passion, which was

---

[52] See Dr. Pawluk's website for more information www.drpawluk.com

[53] Bassett, Pilla, and Pawluk. "A non-surgical salvage of surgically-resistant pseudoarthroses and non-unions by pulsing electromagnetic fields" *Clin. Orthop.* 1977, Vol. 124, p. 117

developing his own inventions. Ed's hobby and rapidly growing knowledge led to industrial engineering positions. He worked in Aerospace Engineering from 1950 to 1983. As his knowledge of electronics, mechanics, and hydraulics became known, he secured steady promotions. Eventually he was advanced to a position as an electronic engineer and section head with the first guided missile plant in the United States. Ed's ability to solve aerospace and industrial problems by inventing innovative machinery attracted several companies over the years.

It was the death of his daughter from cancer in 1983 that turned Ed's interest to advancing the use of electricity for health. Establishing his company, E.F. Skilling, Inc., he continued building electronic devices for electro-medicine, including pulsed neuro-muscle stimulators, the SuperPro, the Photon Genie and the Photon Genius. The U.S. Psychotronics Foundation awarded him the "Man of the Year" award for his Sweep Resonator. Today his company is called the Skilling Institute.

He was the first to build on the frequency research of Royal Raymond Rife after his work had been dropped in the 1950s. In 1988, Ed attended a meeting during a conference in Los Angeles, where several medical doctors showed interest in applying Rife's work with frequency to cure AIDS. Rife had used high frequencies in the radio wave range to kill a variety of viruses associated with specific diseases. Ed had been researching frequency devices so he volunteered to further develop Rife's work to develop a frequency generator.

Ed had also studied the work of Georges Lakhovsky. Lakhovsky had worked with hospitals in the application of frequency in the 1920s. Lakhovsky recognized that cells have a natural frequency that keeps them healthy and resistant to viruses and other pathogens. In order to restore this natural frequency, Lakhovsky developed a Multiple Wave Oscillator to produce high frequencies. The frequencies, in turn, produced a broad range of harmonic frequencies.

When an object is exposed to its natural frequency it will pick up or resonate with that frequency. This is what happens when two violins have been precisely tuned. If the string on one violin is plucked or vibrated, the same string on the other violin will start to vibrate as well. When exposed to the harmonics produced by Lakhovsky's Multiple Wave Oscillator, the cells could pick up their natural frequency with the results that their strength and health would be improved.

In a *Radio News* magazine article published in February 1925, Lakhovsky wrote: "In conclusion I wish to call attention of the reader to the fact that I have obtained very conclusive results not only with a wavelength of two meters, but with longer and shorter wavelengths. The main thing is to produce the greatest number of harmonics possible."[54]

Skilling devoted his talents and genius to the design of a unit incorporating the research of Lakhovsky and Rife to produce a healing frequency and also a broad range of harmonic frequencies. Skilling does not strive toward developing units for specific diseases. Rather, he designed a unit to output **728 Hz** which is the Rife frequency considered to be the most healing. This frequency is carried on a radio frequency wave to transport it to the body. This works in the same way a radio transmitter carries the signal for a particular radio station so it can be received by a radio in any given area. Skilling's unit operates with a very gentle 100 milliwatts of power, a lot less intense than its Rife cousin. The carrier wave of 28.322 MHz is in the high radio frequency (RF) band. The 728 Hz modulates the 28.322 MHz to create a great range of harmonic frequencies - up into the gigahertz range.

The cells can then pick up their resonant healthy frequency. The immune system can gradually grow in strength, thus allowing the body to heal itself naturally rather than creating an artificial homeostasis through the use of frequencies. Ed's unit became known as the RF Flat Pack. The design has since been improved and is now known as the Photon Genie.

Ed has worked with a number of health practitioners who have found that the Photon Genie assists the body in at least two ways: 1.) Increased blood circulation, and 2.) Improved lymph flow.

Ed Skilling has actively lectured and educated America about the positive effects of energetic medicine. Even after gaining international recognition for his work with frequencies, he still selflessly carried on his research for the greater benefit of the Energy Medicine community.[55]

---

[54] See entire article in the Appendix
[55] More information is available at www.edskilling.com

Alexis Guy Obolensky

In the early 1960's, Alexis Guy Obolensky learned about mitogenic radiation from a fellow schoolmate who worked as a Bell Laboratories technician. His work involved the early development of advanced parametric receiving circuits for radio astronomy. One of these uniquely sensitive receivers was used to identify the mitogenic wavelength associated with normal (healthy) cell division, hence the name "mitogenic radiation," following Gurwitsch's research. Over two decades passed before Obolensky was able to apply this learning to reconstruct a viable mitogenic wave therapeutic machine. His "Mitogenic Therapy" paper outlines this work to set the stage for a later "Medical Update" paper.[56] It provides medical histories of routine cancer remissions, as well as multiple myeloma previously considered incurable and fatal. In addition to one documented cure of hepatitis C also considered incurable and fatal. For those professionals wishing to peruse this subject, the participant's names, addresses and medical reports are available.

Obolensky says, "Our body appears to possess a well-defined material nature that changes very slowly, whereas, on the atomic level we are different every microsecond. The majority of our living cells are constantly dying and being replaced. Even the most basic DNA is subject to this continuous regeneration process. The pancreas reproduces most of its cells every day. The cells of the stomach lining are reproduced every three days. White blood cells are renewed every ten days. The skin is renewed every four weeks. Our heart beats 100,000 times every day as we take over 25,000 breaths to re-oxygenate our blood. Today we know the individual cells can exchange information globally (i.e., instantaneously) through entangled-photon emission. Our body essentially renews itself completely every four years. The medical significance of mitogenic waves and Tesla's surviving high-frequency impulse-wave apparatus was not understood."[57]

---

[56] Both papers are available from Natural Energy Institute, PO Box 345, Tuxedo, NY 10987. His email is naturalenergy@optonline.net
[57] Obolensky, A.G. "Early Cancer Therapies Were Based on Mitogenic Radiation," 2003, available from Natural Energy Institute

Over the years, Obolensky perfected a room-size, million-volt Tesla electrotherapy machine that uses a Wardenclyffe-style dome[58] for a crown (toroid) covered in felt in a steam-filled environment. The axis of the Tesla coil is *horizontal*, so that the dome faces the subject, who sits on a wooden stool on top of an insulated platform, usually in the dark. As reported to the Whole Person Healing Summit in 2005,[59] doctors and patients have experienced blue streamers of plasma, different than a spark discharge, that come from the dome (six to ten feet away) and connect to a weak part of the body. In a few cases, the streamers have identified areas containing cancer and several terminal patients have had reversals of their disease. Detoxification is usually found to be helpful in between treatments, consisting of a few days of rest and lots of liquids. Experimental treatments, usually with medical referral, often involve several weeks.

Ralph Suddath

In 2003, Ralph Suddath told an audience at the IRI Tesla Conference and Exhibition (DVDs available) that he had a motorcycle accident which had wrecked his leg so bad that gangrene had set in and the doctors wanted to amputate. Eager for any alternative, he found Ryn Raevis (also a 2003 Tesla Conference presenter) who cured him with an Accuscope/Myopulse device (see Appendix). Afterwards, Ralph was so impressed that he developed the Novalite machine (www.novalite.com) which consists of a high voltage Tesla coil and noble gas tubes, similar to the Photon Genius, to help others experience health and healing benefits as he had from EM frequency baths. The Novalite 3000 can be used in the living room for example, with a built-in timer, and is fairly quiet as well.

In 2007 and 2009, Ralph extended his electromagnetic field expertise to the area of water treatment and obtained two patents on a Fluid Treatment Apparatus that uses magnets and a frequency generator to purify water (US 7,238,289 and 7,473,374).

---

[58] See Valone, Thomas. *Harnessing the Wheelwork of Nature: Tesla's Science of Energy*, Adv. Unlim. Press, 2003 for Wardenclyffe Tower info.

[59] See www.wholepersonhealing.com for more information or contact Meredith Weber, 103 MRL, University Park, PA 16802 for the Proceedings Volume of the WPH Summit 2005. Email: maw9@psu.edu

Chapter 2. Coherent Natural and Stimulated Biophoton Emission

In 1922, the Russian doctor and histologist Alexander (Gurwitsch) Gurvich (1874-1954) and his wife discovered that living cells separated by quartz glass were still able to communicate vital-cell information. Numerous experiments suggested that even some disease was transmitted by invisible light waves in a UV frequency spectrum passed by quartz and stopped by window glass.[60] Dr. Gurvich coined the phrase "mitogenic" or "mitotic" wave since it was observed during enzymatic reactions and mitosis. "Gurvich determined that muscle tissue, cornea, blood and nerves are all transmitters of this special energy."[61] His work is the first

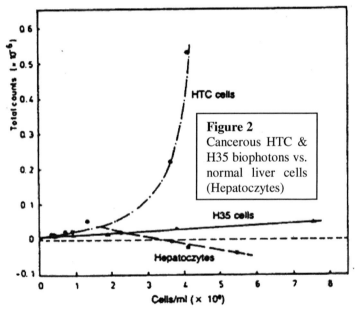

Figure 2
Cancerous HTC & H35 biophotons vs. normal liver cells (Hepatoczytes)

documented evidence of "biophotons," coherent light emitted by animal and plant cells, and became the basis for the design of later bioelectromagnetic therapy devices. It was not until the early 1960's

---

[60] Note that visible light is actually EM radiation in the range above terahertz, called "petahertz" (10^{15} Hz)

[61] Manning, Clark A. and L. J. Vanrenen, *Bioenergetic Medicines East and West*, North Atlantic Books, Berkeley, 1988, p. 43

that Leningrad State University succeeded in capturing the mitogenic rays with sensitive photomultipliers.[62]

In 1976, Bernard Ruth rediscovered evidence of a very weak but permanent photon emission from living tissue, while doing research for his doctoral dissertation.[63] The findings of his research team led by Fritz Albert Popp, subsequently proved experimentally that biophotons exhibit multimode coherent *properties akin to laser light* and not merely spontaneous chemiluminescence which is chaotic.[64]

One example is the unusually high transparency of tissue to biophoton light. It is an interesting phenomenon, which coincides with "light piping" in plant tissues, by which nature apparently

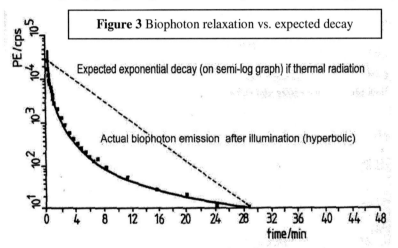

Figure 3 Biophoton relaxation vs. expected decay

Expected exponential decay (on semi-log graph) if thermal radiation

Actual biophoton emission after illumination (hyperbolic)

ensures that several centimeters of cellular cytoplasm do not attenuate the amplitude of biophoton intensity. Experimental data of the extinction coefficient of wet sea sand and soya cells at 550 nm from a Guilford spectrophotometer, compared to biophotons emitted by cucumber seedlings passing through the same sand and soya, reveal the lowest value (extinction coef. $E/d = 0.2/mm$) for the

[62] Douglass, W. C. *Into the Light—The Exciting Story of the Life-Saving Breakthrough Therapy of the Age*, Second Opinion, Atlanta, 1996, p. 269

[63] Ruth, Bernard. "Experimenteller Nachweis ultrawacher Photonemission aus biologischen Systemen" *Dissertation*, University of Marburg, 1977

[64] Popp, F.A., "Evolution as Expansion of Coherent States," *The Interrelationship Between Mind and Matter*, Center for Frontier Sciences, Temple University, Philadelphia, 1992, p. 257

biophotons passing through 5 mm of soya cell cultures.[65] This extraordinary transparency to biophotons inside the body suggests a well-developed *biophysical hypothesis:* **biogenic, long-distance intercellular communication implies information transmission.**[66] Furthermore, each cell that absorbs a biophoton, re-emits it *in phase*, constituting what Popp calls, "<u>coherent rescattering</u>."[67] The total number of biophotons emitted by normal cells, when exposed to sunlight, decreases, not exponentially but with a <u>hyperbolic relaxation</u> of photon intensity after exposure (see Fig. 3 graph). This quick decay phenomenon demonstrates the biological consumption of light energy by healthy cells.

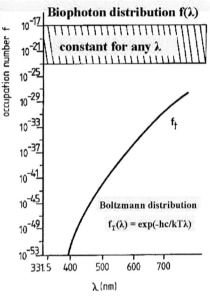

Spectral Distribution of Biophoton Emission

- Spectral intensity is far from equilibrium, able to support dissipative structures
- Reaction rate prop. to $f(\lambda)$
- Activation energy hc/λ provided by biophotons
- **Unlike "white noise"the signal to noise ratio is optimized**
- Coherent photon storage of sunlight takes place that causes $f(\lambda) = $ constant < 1
- **This is a laser threshold**

Biophoton distribution $f(\lambda)$

constant for any λ

f_t

Boltzmann distribution

$f_T(\lambda) = \exp(-hc/kT\lambda)$

λ (nm)

[65] Popp, F.A. "Principles of quantum biology as demonstrated by ultraweak photon emission from living cells" *International Journal of Fusion Energy*, V. 1, No. 4, October, 1985, p. 9

[66] Rubik, Beverly, "Natural Light from Organisms" *Life at the Edge of Science*. Institute for Frontier Sciences, 1996, p. 123
    Also see Fischer, Helmut, "Photons as transmitters for intra- and intercellular biological and biochemical communication – the construction of an hypothesis" *Electromagnetic Bio-Information*, F. A. Popp, ed., Urban & Schwarzenberg, Munic, 1989, p. 193

[67] Popp, F.A. (1992), p.259

The spectral distribution of biophoton emission is taken from Fritz Popp (1985). The function $f(\lambda) = I_\lambda \lambda^5/2hc^2 = 10^{-19}$ mean value, where I_λ is the spectral biophoton intensity (emitted energy per time, wavelength λ, and area). This amazing wideband communication channel should make radio engineers envious. To appreciate what nature has accomplished within your own body, think of a radio tuning dial that picks up your favorite radio station *wherever you dial the frequency tuner*, from one end to the other! It also means that the reception is clear and the volume is the same, no matter what frequency you pick within, in this case, the complete optical spectrum from red to violet (300 nm to 800 nm).

In order for the mean probability $f(\lambda)$ of *photon energy hv* to equal a *constant value of 10^{-19}* (a constant broadcasting volume level) the intensity I_λ has to decrease with λ in direct proportion to the increase of λ^5 with wavelength λ. It does so and the *frequency-independent* biophoton emissions are up to 10^{40} times those of thermal equilibrium and *more potent than enzymes*. Biophoton temperature dependence also has *hysteresis*. As Prigogine points out, Boltzmann's equation is connected with the thermodynamic concepts of irreversibility and entropy, which imply randomness and instability. However, life itself reverses entropy.

Once we associate entropy with a dynamic system, we come back to Boltzmann's conception: *the probability will be maximum at equilibrium.* The units we use to describe thermodynamic evolution will therefore behave in a chaotic way at equilibrium. In contrast, in near-equilibrium conditions correlations and coherence will appear. We come to out main conclusions: At all levels, be it the level of macroscopic physics, the level of fluctuations, or the microscopic level, nonequilibrium is the source of order. *Nonequilibrium brings 'order out of chaos.'* But as we already mentioned, the concept of order (or disorder) is more complex than was thought. It is only in some limiting situations, such as with dilute gases, that it acquires a simple meaning in agreement with Boltzmann's pioneering work.[68]

---

[68] Prigogine, Ilya., p.286

Thus, biophotons are exhibiting a higher degree of order, precisely because of the nonequilibrium defiance of Boltzmann's distribution law. The biophoton distribution is an ideal open system, with the ladder of energy levels, even down to ELF, equally filled with equal probability, like a multi-mode laser, to convert energy not only downwards, but also upwards—a condition for optimum SNR.[69]

What are biophotons for? One explanation is that they are an intelligent expression of the functional state of the living organism and analysis of them can be used to assess this state. According to biophoton theory developed on the basis of these discoveries, *light is stored in the cells* of the organism – "more precisely, *in the DNA molecules of the nuclei* – and a dynamic web of light constantly released and absorbed by the DNA connects cell organelles, cells, tissues, and organs within the body and serve as the organism's main communication local area network. Biophotos are modulated EM waves and are the principal regulating instance of all life processes. The processes of morphogenesis, growth, differentiation and regeneration are also explained by the structuring and regulating activity of the coherent biophoton field."[70]

Short-term (15-minute per day) sunlight baths with bare skin are revitalizing. With the biophoton light storage graphs in this chapter, *there is now a scientific reason for solar phototherapy.* They allow the bodily cells to store light energy sufficient to recharge the *biophoton batteries in the DNA.* Alternatively, exposing the body to a range of optical frequencies from Rife tubes synchronized with HVT PEMFs may also accomplish the same objective. It is interesting that the Azure patent #6,217,604 makes a point of emphasizing the biological advantage of such synchronization of the PEMF and "pulsed light emissions."[71]

The emission of biophoton light by cancerous cells when exposed to white light, demonstrates a remarkable difference (see Fig. 2) in response to overcrowding. The HTC cell curve, representing malignant liver cells shows an exponential increase in activity (positive feedback) with a linear cell density increase. The weakly malignant cells (H35 cells) show a slight increase, while

---

[69] The SNR (signal to noise ratio) for biophotons is extremely high.

[70] Bischof, Marco. *Biophotons – The Light in Our Cells*, Zweitausendeins, Frankfurt am Main, 1995, p. 23 (in German)

[71] See further discussion of PEMFs in Chapter 4

normal liver cells (Hepatoczytes) display a linear <u>decrease</u> with increasing cell density. Growth regulation through biophoton emission follows a nonlinear (proportional to the square of the number of cells) *inhibition*, confirmed by experiment, which shows a capacity for coherent superposition of biophoton modes.[72]

Biophotons have a capacity for delivering activation energy and a much higher potency for regulating biochemical reactivity than enzymes. It is quite likely that the Rife gas tubes of Tesla devices stimulate healthful mitogenic processes and support the resultant biophoton activity.

Some of the electrical properties of DNA are summarized below. To understand how DNA can store light energy coming in through the skin, it is worthwhile to review some organic chemistry.

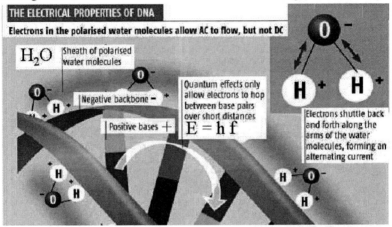

THE ELECTRICAL PROPERTIES OF DNA

Electrons in the polarised water molecules allow AC to flow, but not DC

H_2O — Sheath of polarised water molecules

Negative backbone −

Positive bases +

Quantum effects only allow electrons to hop between base pairs over short distances $E = h f$

Electrons shuttle back and forth along the arms of the water molecules, forming an alternating current

<u>Vibrational</u> or conformational energy changes, of any organic molecule, occur in response to light in the **IR** region of the spectrum (3 − 10 kcal per mole). <u>Electron level transitions</u> of a molecule requires light in the **visible** (40 kcal/mole) or **UV** (70 − 300 kcal/mole) regions, which are of the magnitude of bond strengths and sufficient to excite an electron to a higher energy state, for example. However, double and triple bonds, such as with DNA, increase the chain of "conjugation" and the absorption bands tend toward slightly longer wavelengths. Energy can then be

[72] Popp, F.A. "Biophotons – Background, Experimental Results, Theoretical Approach and Applications" *Frontier Perspectives*, Vol. 11, No. 1, Spring, 2002, p. 25 (also contains graphs used in this chapter)

removed from moving electrons to moving nuclei (vibration) or to biophoton release.

In summary, **biophotons can be categorized as a single carrier frequency EM wave with frequency modulation** (on your FM dial). Therefore, it is likely that single frequency (laser light) or narrow bandwidth light (gas tube emission lines) *are even more compatible with the DNA storage mechanisms,* assuming that DNA's light output tells us what it likes for light input. This actually makes a lot of sense because every DNA molecule is also *receiving* biophoton input signals all of the time. Analyzing the coherence of biophoton signals, laser light is the closest to such coherence, with gas tube emission lines coming in second. Today, both styles of light-emitting BEM therapy units have shown significant rapid healing effects, with PEMF laser devices dominating the sports medicine arena.

Noble Gases Yield Discrete Light

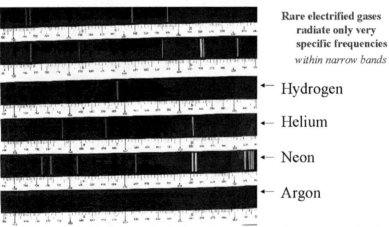

Rare electrified gases
radiate only very
specific frequencies
within narrow bands

← Hydrogen

← Helium

← Neon

← Argon

Above is a selection of a few **noble gas emission spectra**. Each individual frequency line, such as Helium's yellow line (its emission line on the right occurs at 587.6 nm), is known to extraordinary accuracy and precision. Noble gases (helium, argon, neon, xenon, krypton) are inert because of their completed electron levels, making them balanced and geometrically symmetric. They are also rare gases as well as the most stable of elements. Similar to noble metals (gold, platinum, etc.), the noble gases represent great value and attractiveness to those inclined toward esoteric sources of information. Walter Russell, for example, is said to have described noble gases as "octaves of integrating light" related to all the other elements. Single noble gas tubes thus provide discrete, narrow band frequencies for "frequency-specific" effects. Perhaps human DNA knows something about this from a fundamental standpoint since light is stored in DNA.

Is there an intelligence in the biophoton communication method that can be **related to DNA** itself? First of all, 90% of DNA in a cell is not related to genes. When scientists applied two linguistics tests to genetic material from a variety of organisms, they identified 3, 4, 5, 6, 7, and 8-base pair patterns as "words." In the coded region, the words did not decrease in frequency of occurrence in a systematic way. However, in the uncoded "junk" region, the words' frequency resemble quite closely an optical light spectrum and vary "just as the frequency of words in a language does."[73]

In another development, **Dr. Jerry Silver** reports a breakthrough with spinal cord injuries that cause breathing difficulty. Preventing messages from the brain getting to the diaphragm, similar injuries are the leading cause of death in people with **spinal cord damage** according to Silver, a neuroscientist from Case Western University. By injecting viruses carrying the ChR2 gene, which codes for a light-sensitive protein called channelrhodopsin-2, the neurons started expressing the protein. The researchers used pulses of three 5-minute cycles of 1-second light pulses followed by 5 minutes of rest. As reported in the *Journal of Neuroscience* (3378-08.2008), the two sides of the diaphragm started working in tandem in lab animals. Silver conjectures that the **visible light pulses** activates a latent network of neurons that span the spinal column, allowing the two sides to communicate independently of the brain. He thinks the light technique could one day be used to treat people with breathing problems from nerve damage. Patients could be given an implant that would shine light on damaged nerves, eliminating the need for repeated surgery.[74]

---

[73] "Does Nonsense DNA Speak its Own Dialect?" *Science News*, Dec. 10, 1994, p. 391
[74] "Broken nerves are fixed in a flash", *New Scientist*, 15 November 2008, p. 10

Does increased gamma wave brain activity from advanced **meditators** (see Appendix) affect biophotons?[75] Meditation is known to increase lifespan, improve hearing, vision, youthfulness and vitality.[76] It is likely that the gamma wave increase adds to the information communication level of biophoton emission, especially since regular meditators show greater frontal lobe development and less cortical thinning with age.[77] The dynamic anatomy of electrical activity of the nervous system, for example, has already been noted to have a high probability of being information-rich.[78] The mean gamma-band amplitude is the highest frequency brain wave band between 20 to 80 Hz. Long-term Buddhist meditation practitioners self-induce sustained electroencephalographic high-amplitude gamma-wave oscillations and phase-synchrony during meditation.[79] Gamma wave spikes have also been correlated with superhuman feats. Neuroscientist Davidson, concludes from the research that meditation not only changes the workings of the brain in the short term, but also quite possibly produces permanent changes. That finding, he said, is based on the fact that the monks had considerably more gamma wave activity than the control group even before they started meditating. The National Academy of Sciences report shows a ten-times power increase in squared-microvolts from baseline to the meditative state (see Appendix for full article). It has also been noted by the author that HV PEMF may induce meditative experiences in test subjects.

Biophoton emissions may yield a dramatic increase when the brain's electrical activity is correlated to cellular activity.

---

[75] Kaufman, Marc. "Meditation Gives Brain a Charge, Study Finds" *Washington Post*, Jan 3, 2005, P. A05 (reprinted in Appendix)

[76] Valone, Thomas. "Introduction to Modern Meditation, Part II" *Explore for the Professional*, V.12, No.1, January, 2003, p.21-28, online at www.explorepub.com/articles/summaries/12_4_valone.html

[77] Cullen, L.T., "How to Get Smarter, One Breath at a Time" *Time*, Jan. 16, 2006, p. 93 and Phillips, Helen, *New Scientist*, Nov. 26, 2005, p.12

[78] Theodore Holmes Bullock. "Signals and signs in the nervous system: The dynamic anatomy of electrical activity is probably information-rich" *PNAS* 1997; 94: 1-6. (available free online at www.pnas.org)

[79] Lutz et al., "Long-term meditators self-induce high-amplitude gamma synchrony during mental practice" PNAS, Nov. 16, 2004, V. 101, No. 46, p. 16349 free online at http://www.pnas.org/cgi/content/full/101/46/16369

Chapter 3. Effects of Electromagnetic Fields on the Body

While there are numerous other classes of BEM devices, as seen with the Priore machine, the Liboff device, and even pain fighters,[80] this investigation focuses on the High Voltage Tesla (HVT) class of BEM therapy PEMF devices. The standard Tesla coil, with a spark gap between the capacitor and high voltage transformer, sets the standard for this class of high voltage BEM devices which are of particular interest to me. Up until now, the lack of biophysical knowledge surrounding their operation has impeded, in this author's opinion, their widespread acceptance into the medical profession. They are pulsed by virtue of an *intermittent high voltage conduction component*, by means 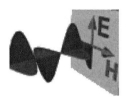 of a relay, switch, a rotary contact, or simply the spark gap, *with square wave characteristics*. To understand such effects, first, it is important to review the literature with regards to common electromagnetic field (EMF) effects. *These EMFs are sinusoidal in nature, like AC electricity.* The electric (E) and magnetic (H) fields are always perpendicular and oscillate smoothly without pulsing or sharp square edges. Such electrical sine waves, if low current, usually have weak effects on the body. However, changing the waveshape to a rectangle (square wave), even at ELF frequencies and in the microampere range, can have profound effects in relieving pain, such as with severe head and neck cancer pain.[81]

Andrija Puharich, M.D., discovered a **cure for nerve deafness** by finding that a triangular envelope of increasing and decreasing audio frequencies, delivered to the skull by electrodes helped rehabilitate the auditory nerves and their pathways.[82] He also patented the invention and attempted to form a company to market the invention but did not stay in business very long. The invention, a Transdermal

---

[80] Maloney, Lawrence. "Pain Fighters—Tests help NeuroControl's engineers design an electrical stimulator to ease the suffering of stroke patients" *Test & Measurement World*, April, 2003, p. 30

[81] Bauer, William. "Electrical Treatment of Severe Head and Neck Cancer Pain" *Arch. Otolaryngol.* Vol. 109, June 1983, p. 382

[82] Puharich, A. et al., "Hearing rehabilitation by means of transdermal electrotherapy in human hearing loss of sensor neural origin" *Acta Oto-Laryngologica,* Vol. 67, Jan. 1969, p. 57 (See also U.S. Pat. 3,563,246)

Model TD-1000, which was donated to IRI after Puharich's passing, remains a viable treatment for such ailment. His complete story is also included in my recently edited book, *Energetic Processes V. I.*[83]

Modality of EMF Effects

In determining the most likely biophysical reactions, this investigation begins with some bioelectromagnetic statistics. The resistivity, conductivity, dielectric constants, etc. of the human body are all known in the literature. There are many stages and possible modalities of EMF and PEMF interaction with the body. Starting from the exogenous (external to the body) field penetration, known interactions with cellular metabolism are now examined in detail.

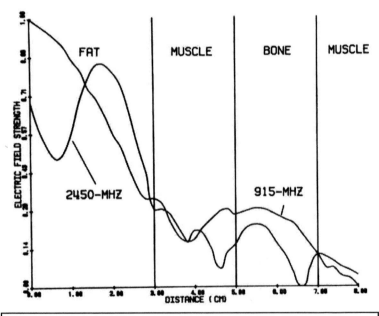

Figure 4 Attenuation of E-field through 8 cm of bodily tissue

---

[83] Moscow, P., et al., T. Valone, ed. *Energetic Processes, Vol. 1*, Xlibris Press, 2002, p. 238

Adaptability of Organisms to Electromagnetic Energy

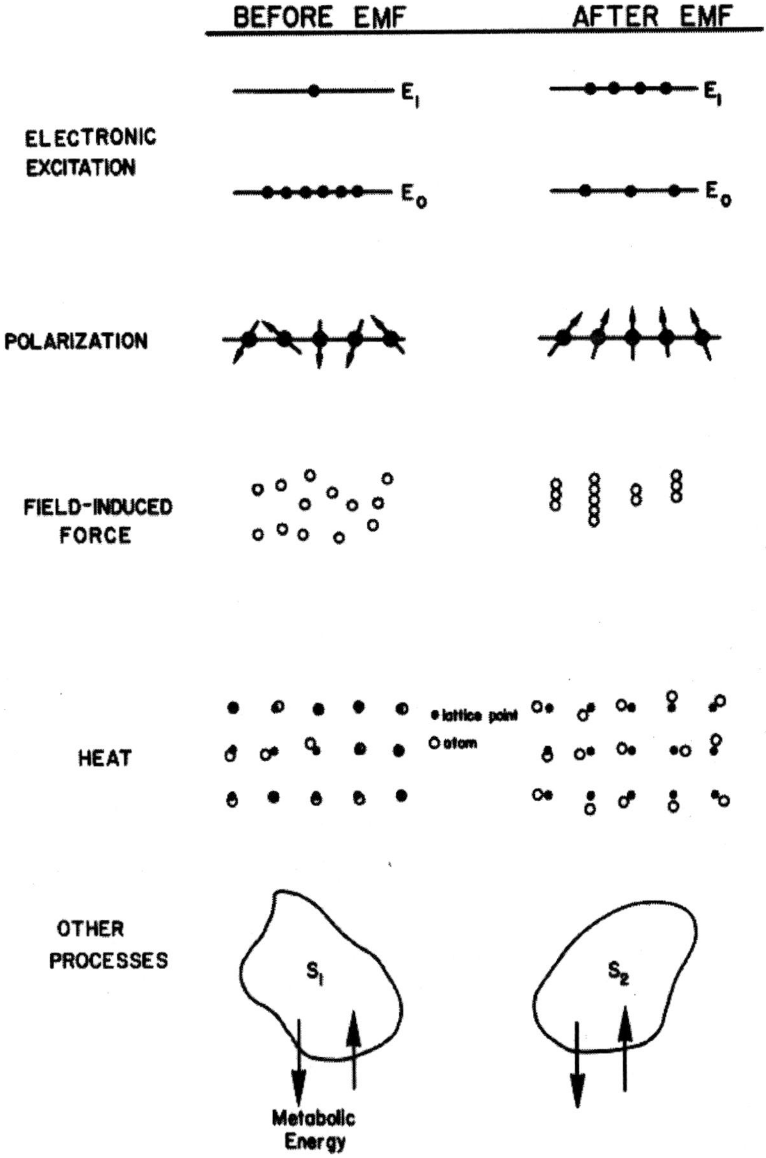

Tissue Penetration of HV EMF

It has been established that low frequency (ELF) or **high frequency (HF) electromagnetic fields can penetrate several centimeters** into tissue, bone, and muscle (Figure 4).[84] Immunological effects of in vivo RF exposure often causes an improvement or stimulation when local hyperthermia is induced with continuous wave, gigahertz frequencies of approximately 100 watts per square meter intensity.[85] However, without local hyperthermia induced, the biophysics of the effects on the tissue is less obvious, so the science of bioelectromagnetics is required.

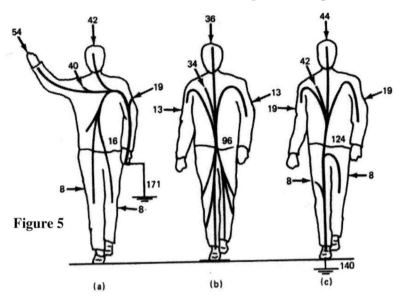

Figure 5

As an example of BEM analysis, Figure 5 shows the induced intercellular currents in *microamperes* in the presence of an electric field only **10 kV/m** at 50 Hz. The diagram shows (a) a ground connection to the arm, (b) an insulated man, (c) ground to foot.[86] An

[84] Polk, et al., p. 281 (source of Figure 4 too)

[85] Ibid., p. 398 (adapted from US EPA, *Biological Effects of RF Radiation*, Elder and Cahill, 1984)

[86] Lovstrand, K.G. et al., "Exposure of Personnel to Electric Fields in Swedish Extra-High-Voltage Substations: Field Strength and Dose Measurements" Biological Effects of Extremely Low Frequency Electromagnetic Fields, USDOE, 1979, p. 85

important implication of this research study seen in Figure 5, as applied to HV electrotherapy, is that those units which apply variable frequency, microamperes of current to the surface of the body using electrodes, may represent only one option for delivery. This is analogous to the story of Dr. Bob Beck (see Chap. 5 AIDS story) who researched the **Kaali patent #5,188,738,** designed to electrify blood with a PEMF signal, which he found could also be applied externally as well (his Silver Pulser), rather than through blood dialysis, as long as the same current levels were delivered. A similar story is well-known regarding the first bone healing electrotherapy machines which used electrodes implanted in the bone fracture site. Later, it was found that magnetic pulsing coil signals (see Chap. 4) could be applied in a *non-contacting fashion* to induce identical current levels in the bone fracture.

Therefore, Figure 5 implies that products like (1) the Electro-Acuscope or the Electro-Myopulse (see Appendix), using a frequency-modulated pulse train applied with electrodes to the skin of injured areas, producing up to hundreds of microamperes of current, or (2) the Silver Pulser of Dr. Beck which produces 50 to 100 microamperes within the bloodstream by electrodes placed on the wrist, may be equivalent to a non-contacting, whole body treatment device consisting of a Tesla-style HV PEMF design.

In other words, the HV PEMF Tesla devices listed in Chapter 7 offer a dosage of therapeutic, pulsed electric current densities since **many operate at levels averaging 100 kV/m** vertically. Therefore, levels exceeding those seen in Figure 5 are induced in the bodies of

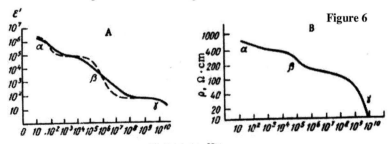

Figure 6

Frequency, Hz

those treated with HV PEMF Tesla devices.

In Figure 6, Graph A[87] shows the theoretical (broken line) and the experimental values for the dielectric constant of muscle tissue in

---

[87] Presman, A. *Electromagnetic Fields and Life*, Plenum Press, 1970, p. 35

relation to frequency for ELF, RF, and UHF bands. It proves that the tissue becomes less and less capacitively able to hold charge in the higher frequency region. On the right is Graph B showing the resistivity ρ of muscle tissue for the same frequency bands. These graphs show, that as frequency increases, the dramatic decrease of dielectric constant dominates muscle tissue response. Therefore, E fields will lose penetration depth with higher frequency ω, as seen in Figure 8. Equations such as $j = \varepsilon E \omega$ and $E = j\rho$ are often used to calculate the current density j (in amps/cm^2).

Negative Ion and Ozone Effects

Tesla HV devices emit ions and trace amounts of ozone which have health benefits, including boosting the immune system

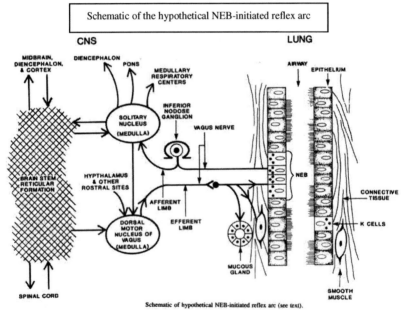

Schematic of hypothetical NEB-initiated reflex arc (see text).

Charry, J., and R. Kavet, Air Ions: Physical and Biological Aspects, CRC Press, 1987, p. 173

48

and killing germs.[88] Since HV devices with a positive ground provide an abundance of negative ions as well as traces of ozone, the graphical *"Schematic of the hypothetical neuroendocrine (NEB) cell-initiated reflex arc"* helps to explain neurological benefits and the pathway of ion-induced effects.[89] The central nervous system (CNS) reflex is quite extensive, with ion-delivered electrons received in the epithelium of the lungs, reaching all of the way to the spinal cord, brain stem and cortex. The traces of ozone assist hemoglobin to bind with a single oxygen atom and thus increase oxygen absorption into the blood. Asthma sufferers can breath easier, with trace (<0.04 ppm) ozone generators nearby, from my experience with EcoQuest air purifiers.

☺ Transmembrane Potential

The *most important* effect from HV EMFs is to charge up the transmembrane potential (TMP). The TMP maintains an endogenous electric field of 10 MV/m (see Appendix & Chap. 5). It is known that damaged or diseased cells present an abnormally low TMP, up to 80% lower than healthy cells.[90,91] This signifies a

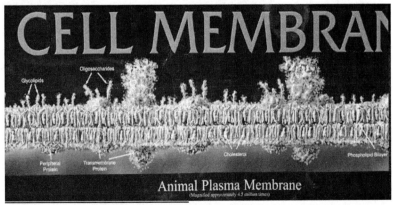

Animal Plasma Membrane
(Magnified approximately 4.5 million times)

[88] Valone, T. F. "Fresh Air Curative Effect Related to Ions and Traces of Ozone" *Explore*, V. 7, No. 1, 1996, p. 70. Reprinted for free online at http://www.explorepub.com/articles/env-pollution.html

[89] Charry, J. and R. Kavet. *Air Ions: Physical and Biological Aspects*, CRC Press, 1987, p. 173

[90] Ceve, G. "Membrane Electrostatics," *Biochim Biophys Acta,* 103(3):311-82, 1990 **Medline 91027827**

[91] Malzone, A. et al, "Effect on cellular and tissue metabolism of induced electrical currents" *Arch Stomatology* 30(2):371-82 **Medline 90314754**

greatly reduced metabolism, impairment of the *electrogenic sodium-potassium (Na-K) pump* activity, and therefore, reduced ATP production (ATP feeds mitochondria). The sodium-potassium pump, within the membrane, forces a ratio of 3Na ions out of the cell for every 2K ions pumped in, for proper metabolism. An impaired Na-K pump results in <u>edema</u> (cellular water accumulation) and a <u>tendency toward fermentation</u>. The TMP electrical gradient is **one of only two ways the body stores energy** (the other is by chemical gradients). This helps explain why adequate TMP ensures that Schwann cells will regenerate damaged tissue without scarring.

A Nobel Prize winner, Dr. Albert Szent-Gyorgi, proposed that cell membranes also rectify alternating currents since structured proteins behave like <u>solid-state rectifiers</u>.[92] Based on these biophysical principles, we can reasonably conclude that a short-term exposure to an exogenous HV EMF potential in the megavolt (MV) range will theoretically stimulate the TMP, normal cell metabolism,

Secrets of Your TMP

- Cell membranes reflect a person's state of health
- TMP = measure of normal cell metabolism
- Diseased somatic and neuronal cells have low TMP
- Micro-organisms only reproduce when their TMP falls!
- Low TMP = Low Energy
  (Low Na-K pump, ATP impairment, increased bacterial & viral reproduction)
- TMP is normally Electrically Charged by Na-K ion pump
- Boosting TMP with an infusion of electrons helps to restore the immune system
- Adequate TMP needed by Schwann cells (replacement cells) to differentiate and regenerate damaged tissue or nonfunctional scar tissue results (Becker, Ann NY Acad Sci, 1974, V. 238, p. 451)

---

[92] Szent-Gyorgi, A., *Introduction to Submolecular Biology*, Academic Press, NY, 1960. Also, *Bioelectronics*, Academic Press, NY 1968, and *Electronic Biology*, Marcel Dekker, NY 1976 (See Appendix, p. 46)

the sodium pump, ATP production and healing. This far-reaching generalization has already been found in the literature: **"TMP is proportional to the activity of this pump and thus to the rate of healing."**[93] (Note: rectifiers convert AC to DC.)

"Increases in the membrane potential have also been found to increase the uptake of amino acids."[94] Healthy cells, according to another Nobel prize winner, Otto Warburg, have cell TMP voltages of 70 to 100 millivolts. Due to the constant stresses of modern life and a toxic environment, cell voltage tends to drop as we age or get sick. As the voltage drops, the cell is unable to maintain a healthy environment for itself. If the electrical charge of a cell drops to 50, a person may experience chronic fatigue. If the voltage drops to 15, the cell often can be cancerous. Dr. Warburg also found in 1925 that cancer cells function best in the absence of oxygen, living on the fermentation portion of the Krebs cycle rather than respiration.[95]

Multiple Interactions with EMF

Some mechanisms for the interaction with EMFs are shown in the Adaptability Chart in this chapter. It includes (1) electronic excitation to a higher energy level following the absorption of electromagnetic energy in the visible or UV spectrum, which is also capable of altering chemical bonds; (2) polarization which, if the dipoles are attached to a membrane, can alter membrane permeability; (3) forces on induced dipoles cause pearl-chain formation for fields above 10 kV/m; (4) heat effects are a "ubiquitous consequence of EMFs" but independent of the details of molecular activity; (5) other processes that have sensitivities as low as one billionth of a microwatt per square centimeter (10^{-9} $\mu W/cm^2$). Such processes include quantum mechanical and classical processes of superconductivity, Hall effect, converse piezoelectric effect, cooperative dipole interactions, and plasma oscillations which are

---

[93] Jorgenson, W. A. and B.M. Frome, C. Wallach. "Electrochemical Therapy of Pelvic Pain: Effects of Pulsed Electromagnetic Fields (PEMF) on Tissue Trauma," *European Journal of Surgery*, 1994, Supplement 574, p. 86
[94] Bockris, J.M. et al. Modern Aspects of Electrochemistry, No. 14, Plenum Pub., New York, 1982, p. 512
[95] Warburg, Otto, "On the Origin of Cancer Cells" *Science*, V. 123, 1956, p. 309   (see Krebs Cycle and Cell Membrane Biophysics in Appendix)

"theoretically capable of serving as the underlying physical mechanism for any known EMF-induced biological effect."[96]

High Voltage Electrostatic Effects

Let's look at high voltage electrostatic fields. Research shows that they have many effects on the human body, most of which appear to be favorable. For example, HV fields in the range of 2400 kV/m (2.4 MV/m) were found to have a **beneficial effect** on mice as measured by their activity, rate of liver respiration, and **ability to form antibodies.** In contrast, mice who were deprived of any electrostatic fields by being enclosed in a Faraday cage showed

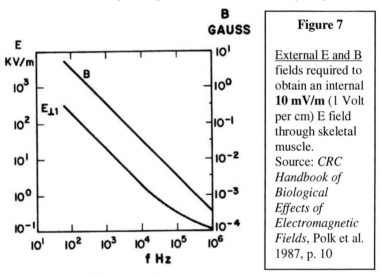

Figure 7

External E and B fields required to obtain an internal **10 mV/m** (1 Volt per cm) E field through skeletal muscle. Source: *CRC Handbook of Biological Effects of Electromagnetic Fields*, Polk et al. 1987, p. 10

opposite results.[97] This can be understood by looking outdoors. The natural ambient electrostatic field caused by the earth's ionosphere potential is approximately **100 V/m** and rises to thousands of V/m during thunderstorms. Figure 7 shows how to create a fixed endogenous E field and Figure 13 shows the delivery system of micropulsations from our natural, earthly HV PEMF environment,

[96] Becker, R.O. and A.A. Marino. *Electromagnetism and Life*, State University of NY Press, Albany, 1982, p. 164 (source for Figure 5 too)
[97] Sheppard, et al., p. 34

periodically reaching 1 kV/m, that matches the requirements of Figure 7.[98]

Endogenous Electric Fields

An example of research with endogenous fields is the temporal peak electric field magnitude of approximately 150 mV/m averaged within the medial cartilage of the knee, when stimulated by a osteoarthritis therapy 0.12 mT coil with 260 microsecond pulses.[99]

In Figure 7, the attenuation of a sinusoidal EMF is shown (with a presumption of constant muscle tissue depth where the endogenous field strength of 10 mV/m is measured). At a frequency of 1 kHz, the body requires an external electric field strength of 10 kV/m to achieve the 10 mV/m endogenous field (ratio of a million

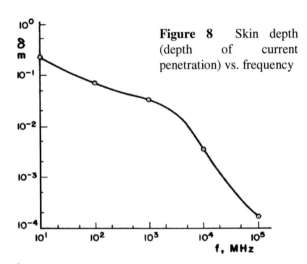

Figure 8 Skin depth (depth of current penetration) vs. frequency

to 1 or 10^6x). However, since the exogenous E field relationship is inversely proportional to frequency (on a log-log graph) an exogenous MHz range signal need only be 0.1 kV/m (100 V/m) to create the same 10 mV/m internally (a ratio of 10,000x).[100]

[98] Valone, T.F. "Electromagnetic Fields and Life Processes" Proceedings of the MFPG, 1987, reprinted as IRI #301 report

[99] Buechler, D.N. "Calculation of electric fields induced in the human knee by a coil applicator" *Bioelectromagnetics*. V. 22, Issue 4, 2001, p. 224

[100] Polk, et al., p. 10

Now to get a sense of the **human body trends** of Figure 7 and 8, we can look at the limits of the graphs. If we extrapolate Figure 7, extending the horizontal axis to 10^9 Hz (1 GHz), it appears to achieve ($\sim 10^{-4}$ kV/m = 100 mV/m). This would then be approximately a 10x attenuation to an endogenous field of 10 mV/m, compared to the exogenous field. The converse for an ELF wave of 10 Hz, is that the <u>endogenous</u> electric field strength, within a few centimeters of bone or tissue, will usually be in the range of only 10 mV/m for an <u>exogenous</u> field of (10^3 kV/m = 1 MV/m (see Chapter 6 for more discussion of Figure 7). **Higher frequency EMFs therefore have correspondingly higher endogenous fields, but lower skin depth,** until reaching the IR (THz) region.

One dependable measure of attenuation of E field intensity used is the concept of "skin depth." It is defined as "the distance over which the field decreases by 1/e (0.368) of its value just inside the boundary."[101] Analogous to the concept of time constant, it allows a range of frequencies to be displayed in Figure 8, showing how deep within muscle tissue a plane wave field can go before reaching about a third (0.368) of its incident field strength. It can be concluded from the data in Figure 8 that <u>100 GHz</u> is a good estimate of the highest useful limit from any BEMs electrotherapy device. Above 10 GHz, the skin depth is only about 1 millimeter (10^{-3} m) so only the epidermal layer of the skin could be significantly affected. Perhaps this would still be sufficient for acupuncture point stimulation however. The reason seems to be the increase in conductivity σ of fat or bone tissue at higher frequencies, which varies from 0.05 S/m at 100 MHz to about 0.4 S/m at 10 GHz.[102]

Frequency Dependent Amplitude exhibited in Figures 7 & 8 can be **compared to an older stereo system**: the higher frequencies might have a their own speaker called a "tweeter" which is small and lacking any additional amplifier; the lower frequencies will correspondingly then have a speaker called a "woofer" which is large but also needs extra voltage amplification to drive the heavy diaphragm. Such additional woofer amplifiers produce the **"boom-boom"** heard from nearby cars today, driven by the younger crowd. Next time you hear such an automobile stereo system, notice how annoyingly penetrating the low frequencies are. That is proof of Figure 8 – large skin depth for ELF and almost complete attenuation for the high frequencies. System science principles like this apply to many diverse systems.

---

[101] Polk et al., p. 11 (Figure 8 graph is from p. 16)
[102] Polk et al., p. 17 (S = Siemans = 1/ohm. Current density J = σE)

Light Affects the Body in Beneficial Ways

Light is a high frequency form of electromagnetic energy that behaves like a wave and also as a stream of particles called photons. The development of monochromatic light sources with single or a narrow spectra of wavelengths paved the way for studies, which continue to show that appropriate doses and wavelengths of light are therapeutically beneficial in tissue repair and pain control. Evidence indicates that **cells absorb photons and transform their energy into adenosine triphosphate (ATP), the form of energy that cells utilize.** The resulting ATP is then used to power metabolic processes; synthesize DNA, RNA, proteins, enzymes, and other products needed to repair or regenerate cell components; foster mitosis or cell proliferation; and restore homeostasis.

Other reported mechanisms of light-induced beneficial effects include reducing wrinkles,[103] reverse eye damage and promote wound healing,[104] modulation of prostaglandin levels, alteration of somatosensory evoked potential and nerve conduction velocity, and hyperemia of treated tissues. The resultant clinical benefits include pain relief in conditions such as carpal tunnel syndrome (CTS), bursitis, tendonitis, ankle sprain and temporomandibular joint (TMJ) dysfunction, shoulder and neck pain, arthritis, and post-herpetic neuralgia, as well as tissue repair in cases of diabetic ulcer, venous ulcer, bedsore, mouth ulcer, fractures, tendon rupture, ligamentous tear, torn cartilage, and nerve injury. Suggested contraindications include treatment of cancer; direct irradiation of the eye, the fetus, and the thyroid gland; and patients with idiopathic photophobia.[105]

Each photon gyrates and bounces at a unique frequency and exhibits electrical and magnetic properties. As a result, their waves are called electromagnetic (EM) waves. The entire spectrum includes radio waves, infrared radiation, visible light, ultraviolet rays, x-rays, gamma rays, and cosmic radiation. The photons of different regions of the EM spectrum vibrate differently and have different amounts of energy, while most are invisible to the eye.

---

[103] Crystal Growth and Design, DOI:10.1021/cg8000703 - Red LED used 90 seconds daily rejuvenated skin by significantly reducing wrinkles.

[104] New Scientist, 13 July 2002, p. 16

[105] Enwemeka, Chukuka, "Therapeutic Light" Interdisciplinary Journal of Rehabilitation, Jan/Feb. 2004, www.rehabpub.com/features/1022004/2.asp

Thus, even though radio waves, infrared radiation, visible light, ultraviolet rays, x-rays, and gamma rays are photons, i.e., light, they vibrate at different rates and differ in photon energy. Their waves have different wavelengths as well. A wavelength is the interval between two peaks of a wave, and relates to the color of visible light. For example, blue, green, red, and violet light have different wavelengths. This difference becomes clearer when one compares red and infrared light. Red light is visible; infrared is not.

Since Mester first uncovered the therapeutic value of red light, different wavelengths of light have been shown to promote healing of skin, muscle, nerve, tendon, cartilage, bone, and dental and periodontal tissues.[106] When healing appears to be impaired, these tissues respond positively to the appropriate doses of light, especially light that is within 600 to 1,000 nm wavelengths.[107] The evidence suggests that low energy light speeds many stages of healing (e.g., 630 nm red LEDs for skin lesions and wrinkles). It accelerates fibroblast proliferation, enhances chondroplasia, upregulates the synthesis of type I and type III procollagen mRNA, quickens bone repair and remodeling, fosters revascularization of wounds, and overall accelerates tissue repair in experimental and clinical models.[108] The exact energy density (energy per unit area) necessary to optimize healing is not critical.

However, there is emerging consensus that accelerated healing can be accomplished with doses ranging from 1.0 to 6.0 J/cm^2. Indeed, recent studies of human cases of healing-resistant ulcers suggest that this dose range results in healing of 55% to 68% of ulcers that did not respond to any other known treatment.[109]

---

[106] Mester, E, et al. "The stimulating effect of low power laser ray on biological systems" Laser Rev. 1968, V.1, No.3

Mester, E, et al. "Effect of laser ray on wound healing" Amer. J. Surg. 1971, V. 122, p.523-535

Mester, E, et al. "The biomedical effects of laser application"

[107] Reddy, G.K. et al. "Laser photostimulation accelerates wound healing in diabetic rats" Wound Repair Regen. 2001, p.248-255

Reddy, G.K. et al. "Laser photostimulation of collagen production in healing rabbit Achilles tendons" Lasers Surg. Med. 1998, V.22, p.281-287

[108] Rezvani, M et al. "Modification of late dermal necrosis in the pig by treatment with multi-wavelength light" Br. J. Radiol. 1993, V. 66, p. 145

[109] Schindl A. et al. "Successful treatment of a persistent radiation ulcer by low power laser therapy" J. Am. Acad. Dermatol. 1997, V.37, p.646-648

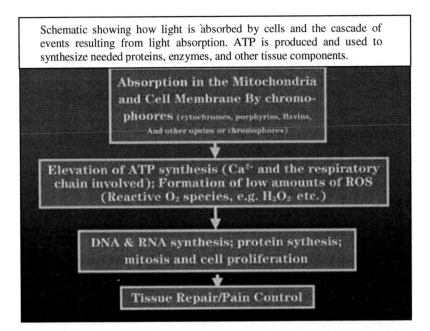
Schematic showing how light is absorbed by cells and the cascade of events resulting from light absorption. ATP is produced and used to synthesize needed proteins, enzymes, and other tissue components.

Absorption in the Mitochondria and Cell Membrane By chromophoores (cytochromes, porphyrins, flavins, And other opsins or chromophores)

↓

Elevation of ATP synthesis (Ca^{2+} and the respiratory chain involved); Formation of low amounts of ROS (Reactive O_2 species, e.g. H_2O_2 etc.)

↓

DNA & RNA synthesis; protein sythesis; mitosis and cell proliferation

↓

Tissue Repair/Pain Control

Overall, the literature indicates that more than 50% of patients with ulcers that do not respond to any known treatments heal rapidly with low energy densities of light therapy.[110] This noninvasive treatment could save hospitals and the nation the billions of dollars spent in treating chronic healing-resistant wounds each year.[111] Twenty-seven percent of patients with chronic leg ulcers have diabetes mellitus. In 84% of these patients, ulcers resistant to healing are cited as the cause of lower limb amputation, which in turn produces varying levels of disability.

Treating a patient with light adds energy to the target tissue. The amount of energy added to the tissue depends on factors, such as the power of the light source and the duration of treatment. For affordable light therapy, we recommend www.lightrelief.com which combines red and blue LEDs at selectable pulse rates, with an option to add in the infrared LEDs at a touch of a button.

Schindl A. et al. "Phototherapy with low intensity laser irradiation for a chronic radiation ulcer in a patient with lupus erythematosus and diabetes mellitus " *Br. J. Dermatol.* 1997, V.137, p.840-1

[110] Surgue, M.E. et al. "The use of infrared laser therapy in the treatment of venous ulceration" Annals Vasc. Surg. 1990, V.4, p. 179-181

[111] Schindl A. et al. "Low-intensity laser therapy: A review" J. Invest. Dermatol. 2000, V.48, p.312-326

Light, at appropriate doses and wavelengths, is absorbed by chromophores such as cytochrome c, porphyrins, flavins, and other light-absorbing entities within the mitochondria and cell membranes of cells. Once absorbed, the energy is stored as ATP, the form of energy that cells can use. A *small* amount of free radicals or reactive oxygen species—also known to be beneficial—is produced as a part of this process, and Ca++ and the enzymes of the respiratory chain play vital roles as well.[112]

The ATP produced may be used to power metabolic processes; synthesize DNA, RNA, proteins, enzymes, and other biological materials needed to repair or regenerate cell and tissue components; foster mitosis or cell proliferation; and/or restore homeostasis. The result is that the absorbed energy is used to repair the tissue, reduce pain, and/or restore normalcy to an otherwise impaired biological process.[113]

The evidence that **low power light** modulates pain dates back to the early 1970s, when Friedrich Plog of Canada first reported pain relief in patients treated with low power light. But during this period the mood was neither right nor were minds ready to accept the idea that a technology that was being developed for destructive purposes—one that can cut, vaporize, and otherwise destroy tissue—could have beneficial medical effects. Thus, like Mester's findings, Plog's results were met with skepticism, particularly in the United States, where until the early part of 2002, the Food and Drug Administration (FDA) repeatedly declined to endorse low power light devices for patient care.

Works by other groups in Russia, Austria, Germany, Japan, Italy, Canada, Argentina, Israel, Brazil, N. Ireland, Spain, U.K., and, of late, the U.S., have produced a preponderance of evidence supporting the original findings of Plog by showing that appropriate doses and wavelengths of low power light promote pain relief.[114] More recent reports include studies that indicate that 77% to 91% of patients respond positively to light therapy when treated thrice

---

[112] Lubart, R. et al. "The role of reactive oxygen species in photobiostimulation" Trends in Photochemistry and Photobiology, 1997, V.4, p.277-283

[113] Karu, T. "Molecular mechanism of the therapeutic effect of low intensity laser radiation" Laser Life Sci. 1988, V.2, No.1, p.53-74

[114] Soriano, F. et al. "Gallium Arsenide laser treatment of chronic low back pain: a double-blind study" Laser Ther. 1998, V.10, p.175-180

weekly over a period of 4 to 5 weeks.[115] Not surprisingly, carpal tunnel syndrome (CTS) is one of the first conditions for which the FDA granted approval of low power light therapy.

In addition to the mechanism detailed above, reports indicate that light therapy can modulate pain through its direct effect on peripheral nerves as evidenced by measurements of nerve conduction velocity and somatosensory evoked potential.[116] Other reports indicate that light therapy modulates the levels of prostaglandin in inflammatory conditions, such as osteoarthritis, rheumatoid arthritis, and soft tissue trauma.[117] Furthermore, works from the laboratories of Drs. Shimon Rochkind of Tel-Aviv, Israel, and Juanita Anders of Bethesda, MD, indicate that specific laser light promotes nerve regeneration, including regeneration of the spinal cord—a part of the central nervous system once considered inert to healing.[118]

Light technology has come a long way since the innovative development of lasers more than 40 years ago. Other **monochromatic light sources** with narrow spectra and the same therapeutic value as lasers—if not better in some cases—are now available. These include light emitting diodes (LEDs) and superluminous diodes (SLDs). As the name suggests, SLDs are generally brighter than LEDs; they are increasingly becoming the light source of choice for manufacturers and researchers alike. The light source does not have to be a laser in order to have a therapeutic effect. It just has to be light of the right wavelength. Lasers, LEDs, SLDs, and other monochromatic light sources produce similar

---

[115] Wong, E. et al. "Successful management of female office workers with 'repetitive stress injury' or 'carpal tunnel syndrome' by a new treatment modality—application of low level laser" Int. J. Clin. Pharm. Therapeutics, 1995, V.33, p.208-211

[116] Timofeyev, V.T. et al. "Laser irradiation as a potential pathogenetic method for immunocorrection in rheumatoid arthritis" Pathophysiology, 2001, V.8, No. 1, p.35-40

[117] Barberis, G. "In vitro release of prostaglandin E2 after helium-neon laser radiation from synovial tissue in osteoarthritis" J. Clin. Laser Med. Surg. 1995, V.13, p.263-265

[118] Rochkind, S. et al. "Effects of Laser: irradiation on the spinal cord for the regeneration of crushed peripheral nerve in rats" Lasers Surg. Med., 2001, V.28, p.216-219

Anders, J.J. et al. "Low power laser irradiation alters the rate of regeneration of the rat facial nerve" Lasers Surg. Med. 1993, V.13, p.72-82

beneficial effects. Light dosage and wavelengths are critical. At present, it is believed that appropriate doses of 600 to 1,000 nm light (**red to infrared**) promote tissue repair and modulate pain, where the visible range is from 300 nm to 700 nm. The FDA has approved light therapy for the treatment of head and neck pain, as well as pain associated with CTS. In addition to these conditions, the literature indicates that **light therapy may be beneficial in three general areas:**

1. *Inflammatory conditions* (e.g., bursitis, tendonitis, arthritis)
2. *Wound care and tissue repair* (e.g., diabetic ulcers, venous ulcers, bedsores, mouth ulcer, fractures, tendon ruptures, ligamentous tear, torn cartilage, etc.).
3. *Pain control* (e.g., low back pain, neck pain, and pain associated with inflammatory conditions—carpal tunnel syndrome, arthritis, tennis elbow, golfer's elbow, post-herpetic neuralgia, etc).

Of course, **sunlight** is the most natural source of light, with the largest bandwidth of any light source, from infrared to ultraviolet light. Michael Holick, M.D., Ph.D. reports the following medical conditions which are related to exposure to sunlight:

- The farther one lives from the equator, the higher on the average is a person's median systolic and diastolic blood pressure, for example, mainly from the lack of available sunlight to make sufficient vitamin D (also vital for strong bones).
- The occurrence of multiple sclerosis also doubles in the U.S. above the 37th parallel.
- Protection from other autoimmune diseases, such as rheumatoid arthritis, as well as a reduction in osteoporosis, osteomalacia, and rickets has also been tied to increased sunlight exposure.[119]

In general, light can offer a photodynamic effect on the body and entire books have been written and conferences held about the specific therapeutic effects of various frequencies of visible light on the eyes, for example.[120] "Studies show that full-spectrum bulbs can reduce eye fatigue and increase visual acuity."[121] Dr. John Ott conducted experiments showing that mice living under pink

[119] Holick, Michael. *The UV Advantage: The medical breakthrough that shows how to harness the power of the sun for your health,* 2003, Simon & Schuster, New York
[120] College of Syntonic Phototherapy
http://www.syntonicphototherapy.com
[121] Stein, B. "Simulated Sunlight" *Popular Science*, Dec. 1991, p. 20

fluorescent light were more likely to develop cancer and reproductive problems.[122] Dr. William Douglass states, "Photonic medicine should soon be used for diagnosis as well as therapy."[123]

Photon stimulation of the skin and acupuncture points is also an emerging science, with some of the researchers (see the Photon Stimulator patent #5,843,074) indicating that xenon gas tubes (see Fig. 11, Chapter 4) are the "closest available light source to sunlight."[124] Following the work of Charles McWilliams[125] and Dr. James Oschman,[126] just the application of such light to the skin is reported to have therapeutic effects, especially when skin exposure to strong sunlight is not available.

To summarize, it has been shown that electromagnetic fields in the light spectrum promotes healing of the skin, nerve, bone, tendon, cartilage, and ligament. Light energy is absorbed by endogenous chromophores—notably in the mitochondria—and used to synthesize ATP. The resulting ATP is then used to power metabolic processes as well as synthesize DNA, RNA, proteins, enzymes, and other biological materials needed to repair or regenerate cell and tissue components and restore homeostasis. Light-induced tissue repair affects prostaglandin and nerve conduction velocity. Numerous clinical studies now support such findings in a multitude of circumstances.[127]

Next to ultraviolet, visible light is the highest frequency electromagnetic field energy available to people. Hopefully, the reader understands from the images of the electromagnetic spectrum in this book (such as the first page of the Appendix) that visible light is just another form of electromagnetic energy, which means that it also falls within the realm of bioelectromagnetics. Besides stimulating the nucleus with visible light energy for the essential

---

[122] Liberman, Jacob. *Light: Medicine of the Future.* Bear & Company, Santa Fe, 1991, p. 109

[123] Douglass, p. 33

[124] Cocilovo, T. "Photon Therapy" *Extraordinary Technology*, Vol. 1, No. 1, 2003, p. 55

[125] McWilliams, C. *Photobiotics*, Promotion Pub., San Diego, 1995

[126] Oschman, J. *Energy Medicine, the Scientific Basis*, Harcout Pub., Edinburgh, UK, 2000 and Oschman, J. "Exploring the Biology of Phototherapy," *J. of Optometric Phototherapy*, April, 2001

[127] See "Light Therapy Applications" extensive report by Prof. Enwemeka, NY Inst. of Technology, 2003, Dynatronics, Salt Lake City, UT

communication it does with biophotons, we have also seen that sunlight in particular is an antiseptic because of its UV content. Mike Hollick's book, *The UV Advantage,* cited in this chapter is recommended to anyone who is concerned about short term exposure to UV. The author and his wife go to a suntan salon at least twice or three times during the winter months, specifically for the UV exposure, which the body stores for weeks. It also helps immensely to ward off colds which tend to attack in the middle of the winter and gives a great boost to my spirits, since I also suffer from the SAD syndrome (seasonal affective disorder). It is recommended that **everyone can benefit from a fifteen (15) minute exposure to the sun each day** if possible. We will even go outside in the cold winter day if it is sunny to sit on an insulated blanket or cushion and open our jackets to get sun on our face, eyes and chest. Yes, even a short eye exposure to sunlight is very important too. I have learned to circulate my gaze around the sky with the sun in the middle, especially in the winter when we spend most of the time indoors. It stimulates the pineal gland and counteracts the SAD syndrome. I recommend at least get a few direct sunshine streaks across your retina each day by moving the eyes from the lowest to the highest part of the sky repeatedly.

Besides strengthening bones, vitamin D also appears to play a key role in keeping the immune system in check. It inhibits the proliferation of cells and of course is created in the skin with sunlight exposure. It also protects against breast, colon and prostate cancer. Dr. Holick from Boston University says, "**More people may die from cancers caused by lack of sunshine than from skin cancer**" (*New Scientist,* 7 April 2012, p. 37).

If you are not able to get exposure to the sun, since you live in an apartment building, work in a closed office building, etc., then the noble gas tube plasma lights with a Tesla coil broadband frequency generator are a good alternative and a compliment to sunlight, such as the Biocharger, Photon Genius, or the Novalite (see Fig. 9 and Appendix). It is also suggested that keeping the eyes open and looking at the electrified noble gas tubes is helpful for, among other things, improving eyesight. These are single gas, complete shell atomic light emitters which emit almost laser quality light that seems to have greater absorbability in the body. In the case of the noble gas xenon, it also closely approximates sunlight.

Chapter 4. Biological Effects of PEMFs

Pulsed electromagnetic fields (PEMFs) are also found to be a powerful improvement to smooth, sinusoidal EMF waves, if it is accepted that higher endogenous field strengths (up to a limit) are desirable to induce therapeutic changes. An example is an electrostatic (DC) 100 kV/m field which *has been shown to improve the synthesis of macromolecules, such as DNA or collagen* (which forms connective tissue). However, if the field is interrupted at least once per second (AC pulse rate of 1 Hz), the DNA synthesis goes up **20% higher** and collagen synthesis **increases by 100%**. A positive dependence on the electric field strength is also found.[128]

As a precaution, it is proposed that the minimum **electroporation gradient of 1 kV/cm** (100 kV/m) should be regarded as an FDA limit, though it is not at this time. "Electroporation is a universal, non-thermal, bioelectrochemical

Figure 9 Diagram of Azure patent #6,217,604. "Method for treating diseased states ... using an electromagnetic generator"

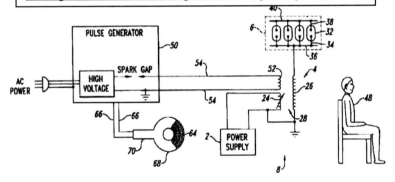

phenomenon relating to the rate of two-way transmigration of chemical ions through the cell membrane, defining the cell's metabolic rate and hence energy level."[129] In layman's language, *electroporation is an electric field-induced opening of the membranes pores*, thus allowing whatever is in the intercellular medium to penetrate the cell wall, including electrical current. "Electroporation occurs as a result of lipid molecules of the bilayer

---

[128] Sheppard et al., Ch. 5, p. 34
[129] Jorgenson, W.A., et al., p. 83

63

membrane to form hydrophilic pores in the membrane…the lipid matrix can be disrupted by a strong external electric field leading to an increase in transmembrane conductivity and diffusive permeability…These effects are the result of formation of aqueous pores in the membrane, which also alter the electrical potential across the membrane."[130] Therefore, any prescription or non-prescription drugs in the bloodstream will have an amplified effect.

In perspective, it may be hypothesized that HVT PEMFs such as the Azure device (Figure 9) and those like it cause a small amount of electroporation and stimulate membrane transport through HF effects noted below, explaining the abundance of healing anecdotal reports. Dr. Robert Adair notes that without utilizing pulsed signals, continuous (AC) RF devices at least need to exceed 10 mW/cm^2 in order to exceed the ubiquitous endogenous noise in biological systems.[131] Dr. Ilya Prigogine, a Nobel Prize winner, points out that *"nonequilibrium wakes them [molecules] up and introduces a coherence quite foreign to equilibrium."*[132]

Concerns about HV EMF safety issues have also been addressed in the literature and also in my work dating back to 1987. Recent experiments confirm that a two-minute exposure to 100 kV/m peak electric field, and a pulse duration of 1 ns "does not have an immediate detrimental effect on the cardiovascular system…"[133] Also confirmed is that "nonthermal biohazards seem unlikely in the ultra-high frequency range" with the chief physical loss mechanism being ionic conduction and dielectric relaxation.[134]

If we compare any PEMF short-term HV EMF exposure for therapeutic purposes to the **long-term exposure to power line fields or cell phone RF fields,** as I am often asked during lectures,

---

[130] Gowrishankar, T.R. et al., "Characterization of Cell Membrane Electroporation" Center for Comp. Sci. and Tech., p.1 (report online at fp.mcs.anl.gov/ccst/research/reports_pre1998/comp_bio/electroporation/)

[131] Adair, R. "Biophysical limits on athermal effects of RF and microwave radiation" *Bioelctromagnetics.* V. 24, Issue 1, 2003, p. 39

[132] Prigogine, Ilya, *Order Out of Chaos*, Bantam Books, NY, 1984, p. 181

[133] Jauchem, J. R. et al. "Ultra-wideband electromagnetic pulses: Lack of effects on heart rate and blood pressure during two-minute exposures of rats" *Bioelectromagnetics.* V. 19, Issue 5, 1998, p. 330

[134] Pickard, W. F. & E.G. Moros. "Energy deposition processes in biological tissue: Nonthermal biohazards seem unlikely in the ultra-high frequency range" *Bioelectromagnetics*, V. 22, Issue 2, 2001, p. 97

the two are biologically different time frames. My professional BEMs experience began in the 1980's during the powerline magnetic field health effect industry inception where I directed a team of technicians and engineers to develop a line of instruments called gaussmeters and EM field meters to measure the exposure level from powerlines in and around the home or office.[135] Therefore, we can state with confidence that **the body's stress response to a <u>short-term</u> EMF exposure affects the immune system in a beneficial manner** (providing frequencies the body may not have stored in a while, which can wake you up), whereas **the <u>long-term</u>**, several hours or more per day, exposure to 0.08 mT (EU and ICNIRP limits for public) or higher AC fields stimulates the body's immune system **<u>too much</u>**. This long-term exposure to high field strength EMFs is therefore considered to˙ be "**chronic exposure**" and can be debilitating (analogous to staying in the cold shower too long or staying out in the sun's radiation too long).

This short/long effect has been confirmed by the **Interphone study sponsored by the World Health Organization**. The 50 scientists involved in the $30 million study[136] with 13,000 participants apparently were not aware of the simple bioelectromagnetics concept revealed above. While the chronically exposed cell phone users (longest time users) seemed to show a 40% higher risk of developing brain cancer, those who used their cell phones *infrequently* had a **lower risk of developing brain tumors** than even those who used corded landline phones exclusively! It's *"as if mobile phones in small doses might offer some protection from brain cancer, which even some researchers involved with the study said made no sense"*.[137] Another article stated a similar attitude of disbelief: "Results for some groups showed cellphone use appeared to **lessen the risk** of developing cancers, something which the researchers described as 'implausible'."[138] The concept that the human body needs a broad bandwidth exposure in small doses to a wide range of frequencies is not hard for the physicist or electrical engineer to comprehend, from

---

[135] See www.IntegrityDesign.com for my original complete line of 2% and 5% accuracy gaussmeters and E field meters (without any harmonic distortion), invented by Valone and sold by Integrity Design and Research.
[136] *Inter. J. of Epidemiology,* DOI: 10.1093/ije/dyq079
[137] "Spotlight: A Study on Cell Phones and Cancer", *Time*, 5/31/10, p. 15
[138] Kang, Cecilia, "Post Tech", *Washington Post*, 7/2/2010

equivalent circuit simulations of tissue, bone, nerves and of course, DNA. However, it appears from the Interphone Study that most epidemiologists and medical doctors have little or no training in these electromagnetic circuit principles. Therefore, such an expensive and well-conducted study offers them only "anomalous" results from their limited understanding of how EMF interactions take place in biological tissue, bone, nerves, mitochondria and DNA. It was a very revealing scientific study, though not to those who conducted it.

Applicable standard for the entire frequency spectrum includes the Tri-Service Conference of 1957 which stated that the incident power density should be less than 10 mW/cm^2 whereas Bell Laboratories (1960) established for indefinite exposure, incident power density should be no more than 1 mW/cm^2 but for incidental or occasional exposure, it could be increased to 10 mW/cm^2.

High Frequency Effects

It is worthwhile to initially examine the sinusoidal high frequency effects. The average specific absorption rate (SAR), seen in Figure 10 for a human body, in watts/kilogram (W/kg), has an increasing logarithmic dependence with frequency up until 100 megahertz (100 MHz) where it levels out at about 10 mW/kg.[139] The SAR for man or rat vary by about a power of ten. In comparison, the power absorption density for muscle per incident milliwatts per cm^2 also peaks at 0.1 around 100 MHz, like Fig. 10.[140] This is applicable to HVT PEMF devices since they operate in a broadband of frequencies (see Appendix), often with two resonant peaks in the kilohertz or megahertz range but still generating measurable energy extending well into the GHz range.[141] HF EMFs in the GHz range (1.8 GHz) have been shown to increase the permeability to sucrose of the blood-brain barrier in vitro.[142]

---

[139] Polk, et al., p. 292 (source of Figure 10 as well)

[140] Ibid., p. 290

[141] Rife Plasma HV Electrotherapy Spectrum Analysis http://www.rifetechnologies.com/Spectral.html

[142] Schirmacher, A. et al., "Electromagnetic fields (1.8 GHz) increase the permeability to sucrose of the blood-brain barrier in vitro" *Bioelectromagnetics*, V. 21, Issue 5, 2000, p. 338

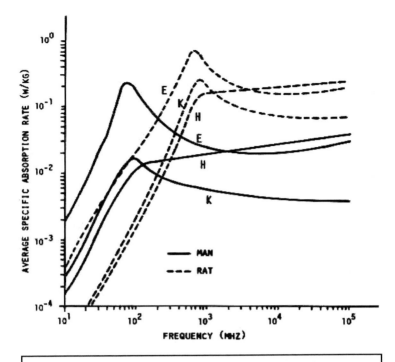

Figure 10 Average SAR (W/kg) vs. frequency (MHz)

Interestingly, PEMFs have rapid rise times, with lots of high frequency harmonics as a consequence (Fourier components), **even with low pulse rate.** *PEMFs therefore, correspond directly to Lakhovsky's philosophy of harmonic-rich electrotherapy.* Experiments on human eosinophils (related to immune system) in vitro used 3 – 5 pulses with electric field intensities of up to 5.3 MV/m and 60 ns (nanosecond) duration.[143] The PEMFs were applied to the human eosinophils, intracellular granules were modified without permanent disruption of the plasma membrane. *In spite of the high electrical power levels applied to the cells, thermal effects could be neglected because of the ultrashort pulse duration.* "The intracellular effects extends conventional electroporation to cellular substructures and opens the potential for new applications in

---

[143] <u>Nanosecond periods</u> T = frequencies f in the gigahertz range (f = 1/T).

apoptosis induction, gene delivery to the nucleus, or altered cell functions, depending on the electrical pulse conditions."[144]

High frequencies in the UV range have been proposed to inactivate the AIDS virus by tuning to the virion's wavelength. [145] **Demodulation of amplitude modulated radio frequency (RF)** energy has been proposed as a mechanism for the biological responses to these fields. An experiment is also proposed that tests whether the electric and magnetic structures of biological cells exhibit the nonlinear responses necessary for demodulation:

A high Q cavity and very low noise amplification can be used to detect ultraweak nonlinear responses that appear as a second harmonic of a RF field incident on the sample. Nonlinear fields scattered from metabolically active biological cells grown in monolayer or suspended in medium can be distinguished from nonlinearities of the apparatus. Estimates for the theoretical signal sensitivity and analysis of system noise indicate the possibility of detecting a microwave signal at 1.8 GHz (2nd harmonic of 900 MHz) as weak as one microwave photon per cell per second. The practical limit, set by degradation of the cavity Q, is extremely low compared to the much brighter thermal background, which has its peak in the infrared at a wavelength of about 17 m and radiates 10^{10} infrared photons per second per cell in the narrow frequency band within 0.5% of the peak.

The system can be calibrated by...a Schottky diode. For an input power of 160 W at 900 MHz incident on such biological material, the apparatus is estimated to produce a robust output signal of 0.10 mV at 1.8 GHz if detected with a spectrum analyzer and a 30-dB gain low noise amplifier. The experimental threshold for detection of nonlinear interaction phenomena is 10^{10} below the signal produced by a Schottky diode, giving an unprecedented sensitivity to the measurement of nonlinear energy conversion processes in living tissue. [146]

---

[144] Schoenbach, K.H. et al. "Intracellular effect of ultrashort electrical pulses" *Bioelectromagnetics*, V. 22, Issue 6, 2001, p. 440
[145] Callahan, P. "Treating the AIDS virus as an antenna" *21st Century*, March-April, 1989, p.26
[146] Balzano, Q. "Proposed test for detection of nonlinear responses in biological preparations exposed to RF energy" *Bioelectromagnetics.* V. 23, Issue 4, 2002, p. 278

☺ Electron Transport and Free Radicals

Many disease states, including cancer, and those called **"aging processes,"** are predominantly caused by **free radicals** in the human body. *Free radicals contain an <u>odd number</u> of electrons* and therefore seek an extra one to complete an electron level. An example is a methyl radical or a chlorine radical. It is known that homolytically cleaved covalent bonds break in such a way that each fragment retains one electron of the bond. Oxygen or chlorine are such examples. **Buy a Shower Filter**[147] because chlorine gas comes out of city water faucets throughout the U.S., unless using a charcoal filtration system. *A home shower is notoriously called "a chlorine gas bath"* by those in the water filter business. Since molecular chlorine (Cl_2) has a rather low bond-dissociation energy (58 kcal/mole) *chlorine atom radicals* (Cl-) can be produced by infrared light or heating to shower temperatures. Once chlorine atom radicals are present <u>in a small amount,</u> *a chain reaction commences.* Each one continuously reacts with another molecule in the skin to produce another free radical, going through 10,000 cycles before termination.[148] **Antioxidants are the most common types of "terminators" for the chain reaction caused by free radicals**, since they offer an extra free electron, which the radical seeks to complete an outer shell. Many types of free radicals exist within our bodies and have been connected with the aging process. An example is <u>acetaldehyde made from alcohol</u> by the liver. It is a toxic chemical known as a "cross-linker" made via free radical reactions, directly contributing to the appearance of <u>skin wrinkling.</u>[149] **Antioxidants are donors of free electrons** and used externally to reduce wrinkles on the skin and also internally to slow the aging process and halt many disease processes, including stomach cancer.[150] Co-enzyme Q-10 can

---

[147] IRI recommends to its members the VitaShower filter which produces a Vitamin C shower for up to two years from the chlorine in the water.
[148] Stretwieser, A. and C.H. Heathcock. *Introduction to Organic Chemistry.* Second Edition, Macmillan Pub., New York, 1981, p. 105
[149] Pearson, D. and S. Shaw, *Life Extension, A Practical Scientific Approach*, Warner Books, 1983, p. 242
[150] Challem, J. "Cancers & Antioxidants" *Lets Live*, September, 2001, p. 76

function as a co-enzyme over and over again as an electron transfer agent or antioxidant.

The electron transport chain found in the body's own <u>Krebs cycle</u> produces ATP through chemiosmotic phosphorylation.[151] It is quite feasible that as the high energy electrons are transferred to ubiquinone (Q) and cytochrome c molecules, which are the electron carriers within the membrane, free radicals may interfere with the process before the electrons reach the mitochondron, thus <u>decreasing energy metabolism</u>. In fact, Dr. William Koch found that "polymerizing unsaturated free radicals of low molecular weight stimulated cancer development decidedly...The free radical formed thus at the other pole...continues the polymerization process that supplies the energy for uncontrolled mitosis."[152]

Electrons are antioxidants. *HVT PEMF devices offer abundant free electrons* to the human body, since they possess a unique HV static field modulated with a multimode pulsed electric field. Such a *flood of electron transfer*, penetrating through permeable membranes throughout the tissues, muscles and the bones, **quench the free radical chain reactions**, since they offer the *very same electrons donated chemically and laboriously by antioxidant tablets*. Clinical blood tests performed by Dr. Ali on subjects of the Obolensky Electronic Wind Machine as well as my recent before and after tests with the Pharmanex caratenoid bioscanner and the Premier 3000 confirm: **Vitamin A levels go up after a HVT PEMF treatment.** Antioxidants normally can only donate one electron from each molecule. Instead, the endogenous flood of abundant electrons from HVT machines can provide enough electrons to force a cancerous *fermentation cycle* production of ATP in the Krebs cycle back into a *respiration cycle* (see Appendix). Cancer cells thus affected cannot tolerate the respiration cycle, as is well known, with its <u>oxygen abundance</u> and instead, tend to expire. The discharging of such toxic residue then will become an important task. "Detoxing is the main side effect of electromedicine, and is the result of the body's eliminating unwanted, toxic waste materials bogging it down. Detox symptoms could take the form of tiredness, headaches, loose bowels, flu-like

---

[151] See Appendix for a detailed analysis of the Krebs Cycle, excerpted from http://library.thinkquest.org .

[152] Koch, W.F. *The Survival Factor in Neoplastic and Viral Diseases.* Vanderkloot Press, Detroit, p. 262 (See www.willamfkoch.com)

symptoms of mild chills or fever, dizziness, increased thirst...all short-term and temporary."[153] When and if these occur, the person should take lots of fluids and only short HVT PEMF exposures with detoxifying interludes. Rife is reported to have used 3–5 minute treatments for his therapy, every other day.[154] Azure indicates a maximum of three 10-minute treatments per day for AIDS patients. HV Tesla devices usually are used even less for all other diseases.

Light and PEMF Synergy

It can be suggested that electrotherapy and light therapy have a synergy which adds more benefit than perhaps the individual parts offer separately. Looking at the Rife HVT PEMF devices which add noble gas tubes to the antenna, it has been shown that PEMF and photo-oxidation together yield "lethal effects on cancer cells."[155]

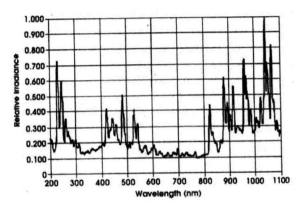

Figure 11   Spectrum of xenon gas

Noble gases (e.g. xenon, argon, neon, krypton, helium) are completely balanced electronically. Their inert character dominates the chemistry for all other elements. Noble gases are also extremely rare in the atmosphere and their individual lines of light emission are extremely narrow, like laser lines (see Chapter 2). Therefore, the human body rarely has an opportunity to absorb the frequency-specific, spectral radiance from such sources in any other

[153] Schramm, J. "Electromedicine and Other Cutting Edge Wellness Technologies" *Extraordinary Technology*, Vol. 1, No. 1, 2003, p. 54
[154] Haley, Daniel. p.116
[155] Traitcheva, N. et al. "ELF fields and photooxidation yielding lethal effects on cancer cells" *Bioelectromagnetics*. Vol. 24, Issue 2, 2003, p. 148

circumstance than with phototherapy devices designed specifically for that purpose. Gas tubes excited by HVT devices shine with easily absorbed, quantum levels of light. Ralph Suddath reported to me that his Novalite improves eyesight if one looks at the lit gas tubes during operation.

Pulsed Magnetic Fields

The development of modern therapeutic pulsed magnetic field devices started in the 1960s, stimulated by the clinical problems associated with non-union and delayed union bone fractures. The early work of Yasuda, Fukada, Becker, Brighton and Bassett suggested that an electrical pathway may be the means through which bone adaptively responds to mechanical input, emphasizing its piezoelectric nature, which opens calcium channels during weight-bearing exercise.[156] Even the National Institute of Health has held a symposium on pulsed magnetic field effects.[157]

Therapeutic clinical studies include favorable effects of **72 Hz** pulsed magnetic B fields are seen in **the synthesis of collagen** by bone cells grown in the presence and absence of the field for 12 hours. The presence of the field even overcame an increasing dose of administered PTH inhibitor, where, for example, at 300 ng/ml there was 100% greater production of collagen with the field present.[158]

Pulsed magnetic fields, often with magnetic coils, has a history of success with various structural injuries in the body, including

[156] Yasuda, I. "Piezoelectric Activity of Bone" J. Japan. Orthop. Surg. Soc. 1954, 28, p. 267

Fukuda, E et al. "On the piezoelectric effect of bone" J. Phys. Soc. Japan, 1957, 12, p. 121

Becker, R.O. "The bioelectric factors in amphibian-limb regeneration" J. Bone Joint Surg. 1961, 43A, p. 643

Bassett C.A.L. "Biological Significance of Piezoelectricity" Calc. Tiss. Res. 1968, 1, p. 252

Brighton, C.T. "The treatment of non-unions with electricity" J. Bone Joint Surg. 1981, 63A, p. 8

[157] www.niehs.nih.gov/emfrapid/html/Symposium3/Tissue_Heal.html

[158] Luben, R.A., et al., "Effects of electromagnetic stimuli on bone and bone cells in vitro: inhibition of reponses to parathyroid hormone by low-energy, low-frequency fields" *Proc. Nat. Acad. Sci*, V. 79, 1982, p. 4180

spinal cord injuries, edema from ankle sprains, migraine headaches and whiplash.[159] The story of Dr. Glen Gordon's pioneering work in Chapter 1 and his coil EMPulse device, approved by the FDA, is also a great example of a well-researched pulsed bioelectromagnetic healing product, to which IRI has added the stronger EM Pulser. See www.bioenergydevice.org for details.

It has also been reported that **a 1 Hz pulsed magnetic field, for 15 minutes a day**, has had so much success with <u>severe depression</u> that the American Psychiatric Association endorses its repetitive Transcranial Magnetic Stimulation (rTMS) use.[160] **Transcranial Direct Current Stimulation (tDCS)** on the other hand, also has become popular recently since it has helped <u>students perform calculations</u> and recognize symbols faster, even six months later.[161]

Pulsed electric fields may also be responsible for the successful application of "earthing" pads and blankets for normalizing sleep (http://www.earthinginstitute.net/), besides the obvious infusion of negatively charged antioxidant electrons from the grounding wire. A surge protector is highly recommended however for protection.

For those with osteoporosis, newer products such as the MagnoPro pad (http://www.omtusa.com/Magnopro.asp), and the EarthPulse Sleeper (http://www.earthpulse.net/sleeper.htm) as well as the IRI OsteoPad (www.OsteoPad.org), are in the market so that senior citizens can access daily bone-strengthening and joint restoring therapy.

---

[159] Salzberg CA et al. "The effects of non-thermal pulsed electromagnetic energy on wound healing of pressure ulcers in spinal cord-injured patients: a randomized double-blind study" Ostomy Wound Management, 41, 1995, p. 42

Pilla, AA, et al. "Effect of pulsed radiofrequency therapy on edema from grades I and II ankle sprains: a placebo controlled, randomized, multi-site, double-blind clinical study" J. Athl. Train. S 31, 1996, p. 53

Foley-Nolan et al. "Low energy high frequency pulsed electromagnetic therapy for acute whiplash injuries: a double blind randomized controlled study" Scan. J. Rehab. Med. V. 24, 1992, p. 51

Sherman RA et al., "Initial exploration of pulsing electromagnetic fields for treatment of migraine" Headache, 1998 Mar; 38(3), p. 208

[160] Milne, David. "Severe depression responds to low-frequency stimulation" Psychiatric News, May 7, 204, V. 39, No. 9, p. 58   and

Arehart-Treichel, Joan. "APA acts on statement explaining principles for rTMS use", Psychiatric News, Aug. 6, 2004, V. 39, No. 15, p. 24

[161] Kadosh, Rol Cohen, *Current Biology*, DOI: 10.1016/j.cub.2010.10.007

Chapter 5. Developments in Bioelectromagnetic Healing

Ultrasound Cancer Treatment Kills Tumors in Mice

BBC News, Wednesday, 29 January, 2003, 22:46 GMT
http://news.bbc.co.uk/1/hi/northern_ireland/2707363.stm

Reuters Health, (c) 2005,
http://www.upmccancercenters.com/news/reuters/reuters.cfm?articl
e=1219

The technique was used on cancerous cells

Scientists at a Northern Ireland company say they have developed a technique that could be used to treat cancer without surgery. Researchers at Gendel, based at Coleraine in County Londonderry, used an electric field and ultrasound to kill tumours in 50 mice, according to *New Scientist* magazine. Gendel said it hoped to begin human trials of the procedure in 2005. "The technique relies on the application of an electric field to a tumour to make it susceptible to a follow-up blast of ultrasound," said *New Scientist*.

"The tissue simply disappears and gets absorbed back into the body," says Les Russell Gendel. "The combination appears to cause tumour cells to self-destruct."

The technique was originally developed to help deliver drugs to inaccessible parts of the body using the patient's own red blood cells. The cells are first sensitised and the application of an electrical field makes them permeable. The cells are then filled with the drug before being returned to the patient. When the ultrasound is beamed, the sensitised cells burst open, delivering the drugs to the right place. Scientists at Gendel found that if cancerous cells were sensitised, they also exploded when hit with an ultrasound beam.

Ultrasound mystery

New Scientist said the technique worked both in the laboratory and more recently on tumour cells in at least 50 mice.

Why the porous cells rupture when hit with ultrasound has not yet been established. The scientists hope the system can be used to treat both accessible tumours, such as those on the skin, and those that are more difficult to reach. Les Russell, co-founder of Gendel, said: "The tissue simply disappears and gets absorbed back into the body."

He said the aim was to produce a portable device that could treat a patient within five minutes. A leading cancer charity highlighted the fact that many potential cancer treatments had shown promise in animals only to fail in humans. A spokesman for Cancer Research UK said the development should be treated with "absolute caution".

Dr Les Russell, chief executive of Gendel: "We hope to access tumours that are not presently amenable."

Listen to audiotape of interview:
http://news.bbc.co.uk/media/audio/38757000/rm/_38757317_cancer.ram

Zapping Away the Blues

SAMUEL K. MOORE, *IEEE Spectrum*,
http://www.spectrum.ieee.org/WEBONLY/resource/may05/0505ncyber.html

Pacemakerlike device to treat depression takes a giant step forward

This month Cyberonics Inc., in Houston, plans to introduce the first implanted device that can treat a psychiatric illness. The implant, when used in combination with standard therapies, can alleviate the symptoms of chronic or recurrent depression in the 20 percent of patients who do not benefit from Prozac, Paxil, and other drugs.

Some 11 million such treatment-resistant patients live in the developed world, more than 4 million of them in the United States. At press time, Cyberonics was working to meet the U.S. Food and Drug Administration's conditions for the implant's approval. A nerve stimulator, the implant is already used to treat depression in Canada and the European Union.

About the size of a pocket watch, the nerve stimulator looks and acts much like a cardiac pacemaker, and it is implanted in the same place: under the skin of the chest. However, it sends electric pulses not to the heart but to the left vagus nerve in the neck. (Typically, it delivers 1- to 2-milliampere, 250-microsecond pulses at 20 to 30 hertz, for 30 seconds every 5 minutes.) The nerve regulates such diverse functions as heart rate and muscle tone in the gut. Two decades ago, scientists discovered that if they stimulated the nerve electrically, it prevented epileptic seizures. In 1997, Cyberonics' device was approved for that purpose. Now 30,000 epileptic patients around the world rely on it. It can be implanted in an outpatient setting.

Early on, some epilepsy patients reported that the device had also improved their mood, adding one more piece of evidence to the longstanding hypothesis of a neurological link between epilepsy and depression. A quarter of the people with epilepsy also have severe depression, according to a recent study. That rate far exceeds the prevalence of depression in people with other chronic conditions.

Phillip C. Jobe at the University of Illinois Medical Center at Chicago proposes that the brain's natural defenses against both seizures and depression are weakened by chemical and structural flaws in neurons that project out from brain structures called the dorsal raphe nucleus and the locus coeruleus and into other areas of the brain. Electrical stimulation of the vagus nerve alters activity in both those areas, although the nerve does not connect directly to either of them.

Six years ago, Cyberonics began depression trials in the United States using the stimulator in the same way as in its epilepsy therapy. Karmen McGuffee, now 34 years old, was among the first patients to receive the implant, in February 1999. She says she had been diagnosed with depression at age 19, hospitalized five times, and given more medications than she could count, to little effect. She often could not concentrate well enough to read or even decide what clothes to wear. One month after McGuffee got the implant, her family began to see an improvement; a few months later, she noticed it, too.

After one year, one of six was free of depression, and 56 percent got some meaningful benefit. Of those who did respond, about 70 percent continued to benefit after two years

----

"I had no idea that life didn't have to have a dark veil over it all the time," she says. "And that you could actually look forward to next week or next month or next year." The only side effect she notices is a slight waver in her voice when the stimulator is on.

More than 400 people with depression participated in the trials. After one year, one of six was free of depression, and 56 percent got some meaningful benefit. Of those who did respond, about 70 percent continued to benefit after two years. But the FDA was initially skeptical of Cyberonics' results, and last year, in a rare move, it overrode its own advisory panel and rejected the device. But after high-level negotiations and the submission of supplemental data in the fall, the FDA reversed itself.

The agency's nod is, however, hedged with conditions on a number of matters, including labeling, the maintenance of a patient registry, quality of manufacturing, and protocols for a study to determine the optimal dose—that is, the right amount of current. Robert P. ("Skip") Cummins, Cyberonics' CEO, told investors he expects to get final approval in time to introduce the device at the American Psychiatric Association meeting in Atlanta, 21-26 May.

The population of potential users of the device for depression is 10 times as big as the one it already serves for epilepsy, and Cummins predicts that Cyberonics will be the first US $1 billion neuromodulation company. He bases his billion-dollar figure on the assumption that Cyberonics will capture just a small fraction of the new market and that its sales will grow as fast as its epilepsy treatment did in the late 1990s. The company's epilepsy business brings in revenues of $110 million per year and is growing at about 6 percent annually. So far, though, the company has not turned a profit, in part because it has plowed so much money into the depression trials.

Cash from the depression business should help Cyberonics explore other uses for its vagus-nerve stimulator, such as treatment of Alzheimer's disease, anxiety, chronic headache, and bulimia. The company also plans to investigate therapies involving the electrostimulation of other nerves. Its patents for such therapies are good until 2011, and Cummins says he expects that they can be extended to 2015.

Besides "talk therapies" and drugs, the only other treatment for depression that is approved in the United States is electroconvulsive therapy, in which seizures are induced by shocking the brain through electrodes placed on the scalp. But the two electric therapies are used differently. Electroconvulsion treats acute, or short, episodes of depression; vagus nerve stimulation seems to work best as a long-term therapy.

Other electrically mediated treatments for depression are under investigation. Neuronetics Inc., in Malvern, Pa., is running trials for a method of inducing current in particular parts of the brain by applying strong, focused magnetic fields through the skull. Others are planting electrodes directly in patients' brains.

Such treatments present a curious twist on getting a prescription refilled. After six years of service, the battery in Karmen McGuffee's implant is nearing the end of its life. "I will definitely get it replaced," she says.

"Electrocuting" The AIDS Virus, A Safer-Yet Blood Supply

LONGEVITY, Sharon McAuliffe, Dec 1992, p. 14

Despite official reassurances about the safety of the nation's blood supply, concern lingers that small amounts of HIV-infected blood may be sneaking through, especially since current screening detects only antibodies to the virus, which can take months to form. But now a new electrical process for cleaning blood of viruses may solve the problem. At the Albert Einstein College of Medicine in New York City, Steven Kaali, M.D., has found that most of the AIDS viruses in a blood sample will lose their infectious capability after being zapped by a very low-level current. Repeated exposure appears to leave blood virtually free of HIV, as well as Hepatitis-without harming blood cells. Kaali cautions that it will take years of testing before a virus-electrocuting device is ready for use. But, ultimately, he predicts, it could be used not just to purify blood, but to treat people with AIDS, by channeling their blood out of the body, exposing it to virus-killing current and then returning it.

Shocking Treatment Proposed for AIDS

SCIENCE NEWS, March 30 1991, p. 207

Zapping the AIDS virus with low voltage electric current can nearly eliminate its ability to infect human white blood cells cultured in the laboratory, reports a research team at the Albert Einstein College of Medicine in New York City. William D Lyman and his colleagues found that exposure to 50 to 100 micro amperes of electricity - comparable to that produced by a cardiac pacemaker - reduced the infectivity of the AIDS virus (HIV) by 50 to 95 percent. Their experiments, described March 14 in Washington D.C., at the First International Symposium on Combination Therapies, showed that the shocked viruses lost the ability to make an enzyme crucial to their reproduction, and could no longer cause the white cells to clump together - two key signs of virus infection. The finding could lead to tests of implantable electrical devices or dialysis-like blood treatments in HIV-infected patients Lyman says. In addition, he suggests that blood banks might use electricity to zap

United States Patent [19]	[11] Patent Number: 5,188,738
Kaali et al.	[45] Date of Patent: * Feb. 23, 1993

[54] ALTERNATING CURRENT SUPPLIED ELECTRICALLY CONDUCTIVE METHOD AND SYSTEM FOR TREATMENT OF BLOOD AND/OR OTHER BODY FLUIDS AND/OR SYNTHETIC FLUIDS WITH ELECTRIC FORCES	FOREIGN PATENT DOCUMENTS
995848 7/1983 U.S.S.R. 210/243
OTHER PUBLICATIONS
Proceedings of the Society for Experimental Biology & Medicine, vol. 1, (1979), pp. 204-209, "Inactivation of Herpes Simplex Virus with Methylene Blue, Light and Electricity"—Mitchell R. Swartz et al. Journal of the Clinical Investigation published by the American Society for Clinical Investigations, Inc., vol.
[76] Inventors: Steven Kaali, 88 Ashford Ave., Dobbs Ferry, N.Y. 10522; Peter M. Schwolsky, 4101 Cathedral Ave., NW., Washington, D.C. 20016	

HIV, and vaccine developers might use electrically incapacitated viruses as the basis for an AIDS vaccine.

Dr. Bob Beck, who was a good friend of mine before his passing, was an expert in ELF, scalar, and pulsed EMFs. He widely published his circuit for electrifying the blood externally without dialysis, thus significantly improving upon the Kaali patent. Two electrodes from the battery-powered circuit are attached to the arm so the blood inside the arm is electrified (Silver Pulser). Bob gave SOTA Instruments the information to make it available to the public.[162] Two products, the Silver Pulser and the Magnetic Pulser are based on Beck's design for disinfecting the blood and lymph, respectively, of viruses, parasites, bacteria, fungi, microbes, and mold spores. The Magnetic Pulser, good for electrmagnetically

---

[162] SOTA Inst., P.O. Box 20019, Penticton, BC V2A 8K3, 800-224-0242 Web: www.sotainstruments.com, Email: info@sotainstruments.com

pushing fluid electrolyte such as lymph, uses a coil to provide pulsed magnetic fields of about 22 kilogauss with a 36 Joule input.

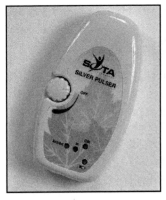 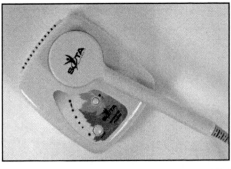

SOTA Silver Pulser and Magnetic Pulser

Nanopulses Tweak the Innards of Cells

Anil Ananthaswamy, 06 February 04, *New Scientist*
http://www.newscientist.com/news/news.jsp?id=ns99994635

A method that would allow doctors to tweak the innards of cells without even touching a patient's body is being developed in the US.

The technique is still in its infancy, and it is still not clear exactly what it does to cells. But initial experiments suggest it might one day be possible to use the technique to treat cancer, speed up healing or even tackle obesity.

The method involves **exposing cells to an extremely powerful electric field for very brief periods**. "The effects of these pulses are fairly dramatic," says Tom Vernier of the University of Southern California in Los Angeles, who will present some of his team's results at a nanotechnology conference in Boston in March. "We see it as reaching into the cell and manipulating intracellular structures."

Applying electric pulses to cells is not new. In a technique called electroporation, **electric fields that last hundreds of microseconds are applied to cells.** The voltage charges the lipid molecules in the cell membrane, creating transient holes in the membrane. The method can be used to help get drugs or genes into cells.

Major physiological event

But the latest technique involves more powerful electric fields, with gradients of **tens of megavolts per meter**, applied for much shorter periods.[163] These nanosecond-pulsed electric fields are too brief to generate an electric charge across the outer membrane of cells, but they do affect structures within cells.

One of the main effects seems to be calcium release from a cellular structure called the endoplasmic reticulum. "In a nanosecond, we cause this major physiological event in the cell," says Vernier. "It's completely indirect and remote, and it's an extremely rapid transition."

The nanopulses can also trigger cell suicide. Teams led by Vernier, Karl Schoenbach of Old Dominion University and Stephen Beebe of Eastern Virginia Medical School, both in Norfolk, Virginia, have shown that nanopulsing can kill tumour cells in culture.

The pulses do not just fry cells, but lead to changes such as the activation of enzymes called caspases, an early step in cell suicide. How the pulses do this is not clear, but Vernier says the effect is not related to calcium release.

Cell suicide

So could nanopulsing help treat cancer? In a preliminary test, Schoenbach and Beebe used needle-like electrodes to generate pulses near tumours in mice. Nanopulsing slowed the growth of tumours in four mice by 60 per cent compared with tumour growth in five untreated mice. The researchers hope that with better delivery systems they could make the tumours shrink.

Beebe's team has also found that the pulses can trigger suicide in the cells that give rise to fat cells, possibly opening up a new way of treating obesity, Beebe speculates.

And Vernier is working with doctors at the Cedars-Sinai Medical Center in Los Angeles to see if nanopulses can speed up the healing of wounds. "We do see an effect, but that's about all I can say now," he says.

---

[163] Note that the normal TMP is 100 kV/cm = 10 MV/m, so the cell membrane is used to an electric field of this order of magnitude. - TV

The next step is to develop a way to deliver the pulses to cells and organs deep within the body. **Theoretical models suggest that nanosecond pulses of broadband radio signals could do it.** "An array of such antennas would create, through superposition of electric fields, a very high electric field right where we need it," says Schoenbach.

A High-Voltage Fight Against Cancer

By Erico Guizzo, *IEEE News*,
http://www.spectrum.ieee.org/WEBONLY/wonews/jun04/0604ncel
l.html

Researchers are trying to kill tumors by zapping them with high-voltage, nanosecond electric pulses

10 June 2004—In the relentless battle against cancer, researchers are now experimenting with a shocking new treatment—literally. They discovered that by zapping cells with extremely brief, high-voltage electric pulses, they could trigger the self-destruct mechanism in the cells' biochemical machinery. This mechanism, called **apoptosis or programmed cell death**, occurs naturally in the body, as tissues continually eliminate cells that are old, damaged, or simply no longer necessary.

The researchers are trying to find types of electric pulses that can trigger the suicide mechanism in cancer cells without affecting healthy ones. They hope the method will one-day serve as a tumor treatment that is less invasive than surgical removal and has fewer harmful side effects than chemotherapy. But critics caution that the technology is clinically unproven and may not make it out of the lab.

The technique's co-discoverer, Karl H. Schoenbach, an IEEE fellow and electrical engineering professor at Old Dominion University in Norfolk, Va., is expected to report his latest findings on 21 June at the Bioelectromagnetics Society's annual conference in Washington, D.C. Research groups in England, France, Germany, and the United States are currently conducting experiments with the technique.

Programmed To Die: Human leukemia cells on a microscope slide were zapped with a single, extremely brief, high-voltage electric field pulse. The cells had been dyed with a fluorescent compound that reveals the presence of enzymes associated with the activation of the cells' self-destruct mechanism. As time goes on, progressively more cells develop the enzyme.

Schoenbach and Stephen Beebe, a professor of pediatrics at Eastern Virginia Medical School, also in Norfolk, first reported inducing apoptosis in cancer cells with electric pulses in 2001. They took mice and injected cancer cells in both flanks—one for treatment and the other to serve as the control—and let the tumors develop. After some time, **using needle electrodes**, they zapped one of the tumors with a series of electric pulses 300 nanoseconds long and **60 kilovolts per centimeter** in magnitude. They found that the treated tumor grew only 50 to 60 percent as big as the untreated tumor, with many cells dying by apoptosis. Since then, the pair has been working to eliminate tumors completely and to do it with a single pulse.

While the result seems promising, it is far too early to celebrate. "This is very interesting science and new technology, but it is far too early to even hint that the method may have a clinical application and, if so, what that might be," says Kenneth R. Foster, a bioengineering professor at the University of Pennsylvania, in Philadelphia, and an expert on the effects of electromagnetic fields on living tissue.

Researchers have yet to perform the many animal and human trials needed to get the technique approved for use by doctors, and those experiments are probably years in the future, Foster says. "There is a big difference between inducing apoptosis in some cells in suspension or in some cells in a tumor and in destroying a tumor in any clinically meaningful way," he adds.

Schoenbach and Beebe's technology is far from the only way to induce cell suicide. Dianne E. Godar, a research biochemist at the U.S. Food and Drug Administration's Center for Devices and Radiological Health in Rockville, Md., who works with cancer causes and treatments, says she "can list about a thousand biological, chemical, and physical agents that can induce apoptosis" in cancer cells and in solid tumors, or that can inhibit tumor growth.

Additional experiments, she says, have to be done if we want to compare the electric-pulse treatment with existing treatments.

One goal of future experiments is to identify what it is in cells that first senses the electric pulses and triggers apoptosis. That information can then be used to find a way to target cancer cells specifically. "There's something that occurs in the cell that it cannot resolve, it cannot fix; so it commits suicide," says Beebe. He says cellular structures known to regulate programmed cell death, including the energy-producing mitochondria and the DNA-storing nucleus, might be involved.

Understanding apoptosis is among the hottest topics in medicine and molecular biology nowadays. The 2002 <u>Nobel Prize</u> in Physiology or Medicine went to three researchers—Sydney Brenner, John Sulston, and Robert Horvitz—for their seminal work on apoptosis and the genetic regulation of organ development.

Problems with apoptosis are implicated in many diseases, including cancer—when cells fail to undergo apoptosis and multiply wildly—and neurodegenerative disorders such as Alzheimer's disease—when too many cells die. So, for cancer, scientists want to find ways to induce apoptosis; for Alzheimer's, they want to block it.

Decades before the focus on apoptosis, scientists used electric pulses of a lower voltage and longer duration to create temporary pores in the outer membranes of cells. This technique, called **electroporation**, is now widely used in laboratories to inject cells with DNA, drugs, and other kinds of molecules.

A cell in an electric field behaves essentially as a tiny spherical capacitor: its 5-nanometer-thick membrane is a good insulator and is surrounded, inside and out, mostly by salty water. When a field is applied, ions and other charged molecules in the water accumulate outside the cell's membrane. The same process happens inside the cell, and as a result, a voltage builds up across the membrane.[164]

"When the voltage across the membrane gets up to between 0.5 and 1 volt, something dramatic happens," says James C. Weaver, a senior research scientist at the Harvard-Massachusetts Institute of Technology's Division of Health Sciences and Technology, in Cambridge. The voltage causes a breakdown in the membrane's insulating properties, opening a large number of

---

[164] This also nicely illustrates the buildup of the TMP.   - TV

temporary pores all over it. Ions and other large molecules can pass through the pores in the membrane, which temporarily changes from being an insulator to being a conductor.

Today, electroporation is used experimentally to enhance the efficacy of chemotherapy, Weaver says that the procedure opens large pores in cancer cells, forcing them to absorb more of an anticancer drug such as bleomycin, which damages DNA, killing the cell. Researchers working on this combination of electroporation and chemotherapy include Lluis Mir at the CNRS-Institute Gustave-Roussy, in Villejuif, in France; Richard Heller at the University of South Florida, Tampa; and researchers at the Genetronics Biomedical in San Diego.

The electric field pulses used in such experiments have intensities on the order of **kilovolts per centimeter**, which last from microseconds to milliseconds. But Schoenbach realized that a pulse with a shorter duration, on the order of nanoseconds, would not last long enough to bring ions to the cell membrane and build a voltage high enough to break it down. Instead, the faster pulse seems to bypass the cell membrane, affecting structures inside cells such as the nucleus. Like the cell itself, these structures have membranes that are good insulators, and **therefore they also act as tiny capacitors that can charge up.**

Schoenbach and Beebe discovered that these short, high intensity pulses could jolt the guts of the cells in a way that activates their self-destruction machinery. So, in principle, a treatment based on these short pulses would not require a drug like bleomycin: the pulses themselves would be the killing agents.

Delivering such a tremendous voltage in just a few billionths of a second is akin to accelerating a car from 0 to 100 kilometers per hour and then decelerating it back to 0, all within 1 second. The system Schoenbach's group built to perform the task consists of a commercially available high-voltage source used in powerful lasers and X-ray devices connected to a so-called pulse form network, a circuit that creates the nanoseconds-long powerful electric field between two electrodes.

The pulse form network, Schoenbach says, is a complex arrangement of interconnected cables and electronic components, but it works essentially as a transmission line. The 40,000-kV source delivers a burst of electrical energy to one end of the line through a spark-gap switch and it travels toward the electrodes.

During the brief time the stream of energy flows along the line—a few billionths of a second—an electric field of hundreds of kilovolts per centimeter appears between the tiny electrodes.

The electrodes, usually a few millimeters apart, don't necessarily need to touch the cells. It is the electric field between them that does the work. So far, the group has used needles as electrodes, but researchers are studying other sophisticated ways of applying the field, including antennas that could zap a tumor inside the body at a distance. "That's a daunting task," Schoenbach says. "We need extremely high electric fields and high power broadband antennas. That's really futuristic at this point."

Regardless of how the pulses are delivered, the high voltages involved make the setup sounds more like a new cooking technique than a cancer treatment. But the actual energy delivered is quite low, less than a joule, not even enough to heat the cells single degree Celsius. This is because, even though the amount of power involved is enormous—16 megawatts or 16 megajoules per second—it is applied for only a few nanoseconds.

" Usually when people think about electricity, they think about a brutal way of killing—electrocution, burning, this kind of thing," says Schoenbach. "Our method is focusing on extremely short pulses, so that there's no thermal effect, no heating involved. It's purely an electrical effect."

Ultimately, the success of ultrafast, high-voltage pulses as a cancer treatment depends on whether a pulse of particular duration or voltage will preferentially kill tumor cells rather than normal cells. "The trick with all cancer therapies is to find a therapeutic window where the therapy kills the tumor cells without too great a collateral effect on sensitive normal tissues," says Gerard I. Evan, a professor of cancer biology at the University of California at San Francisco.

Evan says the results obtained by Schoenbach, Beebe, and their colleagues are intriguing, but more experiments are necessary to determine whether such electric fields would exhibit the necessary specificity. It's particularly important, he says, that researchers identify the molecular mechanism by which the pulses trigger apoptosis. Only then will it be possible to get some idea as to whether the pulses might be effective as a treatment some day.

And researchers have yet to figure out what exactly is happening within zapped cells. "We know the start—we have to have this series of extremely short pulses. And we know the end—we create apoptosis," Schoenbach says. "What we're looking for now is what is in between."

Air Ionisers Wipe out Hospital Infections

Natasha McDowell
January 3, 2003 *New Scientist*

Repeated airborne infections of the bacteria acinetobacter in an intensive care ward have been eliminated by the installation of a negative air ioniser. In the first such epidemiological study, researchers found that the infection rate fell to zero during the year long trial. "We were absolutely astounded to find such clear cut results," engineer Clive Begg at the University of Leeds, UK, told New Scientist.

Stephen Dean, a consultant at the St James's Hospital in Leeds where the trial took place says: "The results have been fantastic - so much so that we have asked the university to leave the ionisers with us." The ionisers produce negative air ions that collide with suspended particles and give them a charge. The scientists believe charged particles aggregate together and fall out of the air, thereby disinfecting the atmosphere and stopping the transmission of infection.

"We don't fully understand how it is working, but we suspect it is damaging or killing the bacteria," says Beggs. "But if the ionisers are cleaning the air in this way, we would expect to find more precipitation of acinetobacter on surfaces and this is exactly what we found."

Antibiotic resistant

Acinetobacter infections are often very difficult to treat as the bacterium is resistant to many antibiotics. It poses no real threat to healthy humans but can cause serious infections in people with weakened immune systems.

"Ionisers may become a powerful weapon in the fight against hospital acquired infection," says clinical microbiologist Kevin Kerr, another team member. "People had focused on getting doctors and nurses to wash their hands and had not looked at anything else." About 10 per cent of infections in the UK's public hospitals have been estimated to be airborne, but Kerr says it may be even higher, as conventional methods to sample airborne bacteria are inefficient.

But although the results are very promising, he adds that further research is needed because acinetobacter infections tend to be cyclical. "They may not be seen for weeks or months and then you see a cluster of infections," he says.

Tuberculosis target

The team is currently doing more lab studies to see if other organisms may be targeted. Tuberculosis is one promising target. Brian Duerden, director of the UK's Public Health Laboratory Service, is encouraged by the results. "It is not the whole answer as many infections are spread by touch, but it is a potential addition to the weaponry against hospital infections," he told *New Scientist*.

Research by electronics company Sharp has shown that positive and negative ions produced by their **air conditioning systems can inactivate viruses including influenza.** But the new study is the first to link such an effect to reduced infections in hospitals. [165]

Electrons are Antioxidants

FREE RADICALS STEAL ELECTRONS
creating more free radical DAMAGE in a chain reaction (10,000 times)

Damaged mitochondrial DNA causes aging

ANTIOXIDANTS STOP FREE RADICALS WITH ELECTRONS

References
• "Oxidative damage causes aging" - *Life Enhancement*, Oct. 2004
• "Dying before their time: studies of prematurely old mice hint that DNA mutations underlie aging." *Science News*, July 10, 2004, p. 26
• "Mice and mitochondria" Martin, *Nature*, 2004, V. 429, p. 357,417

---

[165] Note: Air ionizers use a HV electrical output below 10 kV. Properly designed PEMF devices have negative polarity so that plenty of negative ions (carrying free electrons) are generated. - TV

Chapter 6. Electropulsations Occur in Nature

The earth-ionosphere cavity acts as a spherical capacitor, which capacitively couples with the condenser (capacitor) of the human body. This statement is not just speculation. Much research has been done to show the profound <u>EEG entrainment</u> that the earth's "micropulsations" (Schumann resonances) cause in the human body, as long as the person is isolated from stronger EMFs. The picotesla (nanogauss) *micropulsations* of the earth at a fundamental frequency of 8 Hz, easily entrain the alpha rhythm of the human brain, also centered at 8 Hz, which only exhibits 1/1000 of the earth's AC magnetic field strength.[166] Human magnetoencephalograms (MEG) are in the femtotesla (picogauss) range.[167] As seen in the simultaneous worldwide recording below,

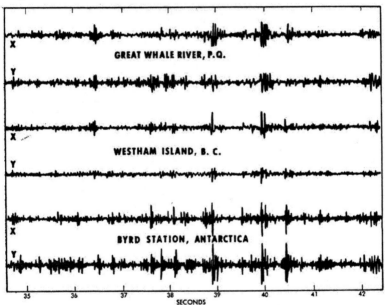

Fig. 12 Earth micropulsations (2 -- 30 Hz) recorded simultaneously. Source: Galejs, *Terrestrial Propagation of Long Electromagnetic Waves*, Pergamon Press, 1972

---

[166] Dubrov, A. P. *The Geomagnetic Field and Life: Geomagnetobiology*, Plenum Press, New York, 1978
[167] Valone, T. "MEG Amplification With an ELF Magnetometer," IRI Report #202, 1995. Also see Valone, T. "Electromagnetic Fields and Life Processes" IRI Report #301, 1991

we have evolved in a PEMF environment, more specifically a resonant electromagnetic cavity shaped like a spherical shell, with the earth's 24-hour electromagnetic pulses naturally impinging on our brain, body and nervous system. You can listen to these VLF "earth songs" at a NASA website as well.[168] "These oscillations are excited by naturally occurring lightning discharges..."[169] *HV static and dynamic EMFs have been an integral part of the human experience for thousands of years of evolution* so that we biologically thrive in response to them. Interestingly, all of the laboratory "synthesis of life" (origin of life) experiments also use electric discharge (spark or corona), UV radiation, heat or ionizing radiation to stimulate the production of amino acids from basic building blocks.[170]

Below is the compilation of the earth's micropulsations.[171] Comparing this graph to the declining E and B fields of Figure 7, it has the same slope. Therefore, *the earth-ionosphere cavity must deliver a fixed amplitude of its pulsating E field inside the human body, estimated to be 1-10 pV/m, independent of frequency.*[172]

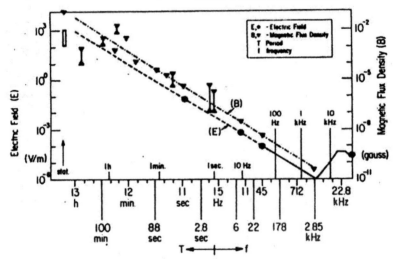

Figure 13   Earth Schumann cavity E and B fields from 0 to 50 kHz

---

[168] Earth VLF Sounds: http://www.spaceweather.com/glossary/inspire.html
[169] Galejs, J., p. 241
[170] Price, C.C. *Synthesis of Life*, Dowden, Hutchison & Ross, 1974, p.24
[171] Persinger, M. ed., *ELF and VLF EMF Effects*, Plenum, NY, 1974, p. 14
[172] Prove it using E=2πfBr/2 with r = 0.1m & Fig. 13-14 data (B in Tesla).

This also can also be verified with Figures 13 and 14 data considering Faraday's law, since the earth's cavity micropulsation B field is seen to be <u>inversely proportional to frequency</u>. *It is nature's predecessor to spread spectrum communications.*

> **21st Century Gaia Principle:** *The earth is intimately linked by wideband electromagnetic communications with biological life. Humans, etc. are like radios with the same reception and sound level across all the frequency bands.*

Furthermore, the endogenous fixed pV/m amplitude of the external cavity oscillations, being independent of frequency, is also analogous to the behavior of the "f(λ)= constant" rule of biophotons, in Chapter 2. That is, *while cell biophotons <u>broadcast</u> with equal amplitude across all frequencies,* **the body also <u>receives</u> the earth's atmospheric cavity broadcast, just like biophoton reception,** *equally well at any available broadcast frequency.*

To increase the amplitude of earthly micropulsations worldwide would thus be biologically beneficial, and already been proposed.[173]

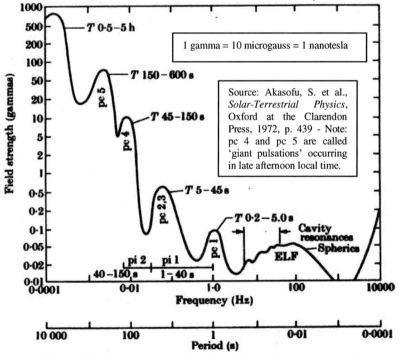

Figure 14 Geomagnetic pulsations of earth-ionosphere cavity

---

[173] Valone, T. *Harnessing the Wheelwork of Nature*, Adventures Unlimited, 2002, p. 89 - 270

Chapter 7. Summary and Conclusion

To summarize the main findings presented in this book, the following points are duly emphasized:

- High voltage electrotherapy **PEMF machines** have a 100-year history of success, with surprisingly **few side effects**;
- **Light exposure directly to the skin** has numerous energy-recharging effects, increasing ATP – get some sun each day;
- **Beneficial biological effects** of short-term exposure to EMFs include HV effects, PEMF effects, ion/ozone effects, and most importantly, *TMP stimulation and restoration*;
- **HV EMFs** penetrate the body easily, inducing <u>microamperes</u> of intercellular electron and ion flow;
- **Cell membranes** are known to **rectify EMFs** and are capable of <u>demodulation of all EMFs</u> with biophotons as optical EMFs, which aids in explaining **information transfer**;
- **Tesla HV PEMF devices induce a flood of electrons which are antioxidants** that penetrate the clothing and skin, *terminating free radicals* and thus, slowing the aging process;
- **E & B earth field** log-log graphs[174] show a linear, inverse proportionality with frequency but constant endogenous E-field
- **Body cells *broadcast* biophotons** with equal probability across all frequencies and also ***receive*** earth's atmospheric cavity EMFs and broadband cellular biophotons, <u>both</u> without preference for frequency, maximizing information transfer;
- **HVT PEMF devices**, near to the human body, **increase ATP production levels** in the cells due to the abundance of energetic electrons, and *feed the healthful respiration portion of the Krebs cycle*, rather than the cancerous fermentation portion;
- **BEMs healing effect** by HVT PEMFs can be mainly correlated to the **1) optimization of the Na-K pump** in the cells' membranes and **2) the increase in the TMP** <u>which boosts the immune system.</u>
- <u>Brief broadband PEMF bath a day</u> helps keep the doctor away.

---

[174] A graph with logarithms plotted on both axes shows a straight line for a double exponential equation where terms on both sides of the equation have exponents.

In conclusion, the PEMF devices that are known to utilize a Tesla coil, for the HF and HV PEMF, include the Azure patent (US Patent #6,217,604), the Novalite Machine (www.novalite.com), the PREMIER Jr. (www.IntegrityResearchInstitute.org), the Biocharger (www.biocharger.com), the Light Beam Generator (www.LightBeamGenerator.com), the Lakhovsky multiwave oscillator (MWO) (www.BioEnergyDevice.org), and the Rejuvematrix (www.NormShealy.com). Several of these also add biophoton-stimulating high voltage gas tubes following Rife's design which benefit the body. We caution against large magnetic field coils that can also induce powerful PEMF currents, such as the PAP IMI (US Patent #5,068,039 and #5,556,418) since the strong electroporation can increase absorption of drugs and chemicals in the blood. Deleterious side effects are reported from PAP IMI use.

Table of EMF Studies & Statistics Cited in Text

E = electric field (AC unless indicated); B = magnetic field (AC unless indicated); Hz = frequency in Hertz

EXTERNAL INPUT	INDUCED RESULT IN THE BODY - endogenous EM field effects -	Pg
100-1000 V/m @ 0.0001Hz – 50 kHz	1-10 picovolts/meter constant amplitude of entire band in tissues of everyone on a daily basis	90
10 kV/m E	Up to 170 µA in intercellular fluid and tissue	46
10 kV/m @ 1kHz	10 mV/m inside muscle tissue	52
100 kV/m static E	Improved synthesis of DNA and collagen	62
100 kV/m @ 1Hz	100% better collagen synthesis than static E	63
100kV/m for 1ns	Pulses had no effect on cardiovascular system	64
1 MV/m @ 10 Hz	10 mV/m inside muscle tissue (Fig. 7)	52
2.4 MV/m static E	Liver respiration and antibody improvement	52
5.3 MV/m for 60ns	No permanent disruption of plasma membrane	67
10 MV/m	Transmembrane electric potential	49
----------------------	---	----
0.12 mT custom B	150 mV/m with 0.26 ms pulse width inside knee	53
"	3 mV @ 16 Hz and 5 – 20 µA inside bone	129
B pulsed @ 72 Hz	Favorable synthesis of collagen - bone cells; 12 hrs	72
100 MHz	0.1 m (100 cm) skin depth of penetration (Fig. 8)	53
1 – 2 GHz	Penetrates up to 8 cm of mixed tissue (Fig. 4)	44
1.8 GHz	Sucrose permeability inc. in blood-brain barrier	67
mW/cm^2 @ MHz	10 mW/kg average human absorption (Fig. 10)	66
1 mW/cm^2@100MHz	SAR of 0.1 - absorbed in muscle tissue (Fig. 10)	66
10 mW/cm^2	Minimum to exceed endogenous noise	64
100 W/m^2 @ GHz	Favorable immunological effects (=10 mW/cm^2)	46

APPENDIX

Bioelectromagnetic Healing

Resources and Reference Material

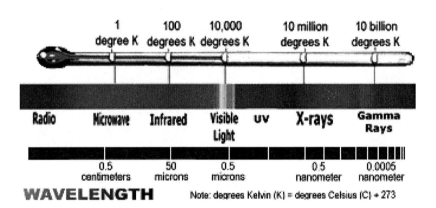

Cell Membrane Biophysics

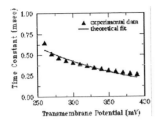

Transmembrane Activity

- Molecular transport by active and passive means
- Energy mediates the active transport mode
- TMP is at least 100 mV across 1 nm lipid bilayer
- TMP therefore can withstand 100 kV/cm (10x air!)
- Electroporation happens in the range of 1 kV/cm

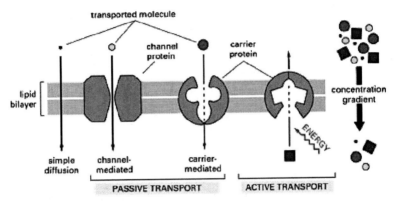

Here "ENERGY" is indicated in the Active Transport as an option for the membrane pore to open and allow active transport of nutrients and or electrons from the intercellular fluid. Such energy can be provided in many ways including by electromagnetic fields. EMF interactions are seen on the next page in the "Lipo-protein Soliton Interactions" diagram.[175] impinging on the left side of the extracellular portion (outside) of the membrane. The lipo-protein has a polar end with + on the upper part and – on the lower, membrane lipid part, constituting a rectifier. This is basically what motivated A. Szent-Gyorgi concerning rectified (DC) EMFs inside the cell upon (AC) EMFs perturbing the extracellular surface.

Interestingly enough, researchers have proposed equivalent circuits for biological membranes to work out the response to EMF perturbations. With such a circuit, pictured on the next page, and parameters verified by experiment, it is easier to imagine "the

---

[175] Adey, W.R. "Nonlinear, nonequilibrium aspects of electromagnetic field interactions at cell membranes" *Nonlinear Electrodynamics in Biological Systems*, Plenum Press, New York, 1985, p. 17

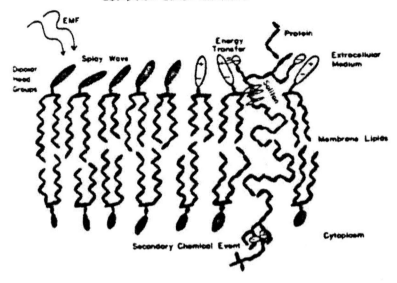

Lipo-protein Soliton Interactions

possibility of electron transfer as a result of artificial change in potential" which amounts to a current flow across the cell membrane.[176] In response to the EMF perturbation, Pilla explains that the first response will be a current flow, assuming that it can respond in a linear fashion with $I(t) = dq/dE \, (dn/dt)$ where q is the interfacial charge, E is the unperturbed potential (volts) across the membrane, and n is the change in potential due to the EMF.

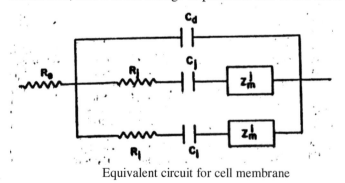

Equivalent circuit for cell membrane

---

[176] Pilla, Arthur. "Electrochemical Information Transfer at Living Cell Membranes" *Annals of the NY Academy of Science*, V. 238, 1974, p. 149

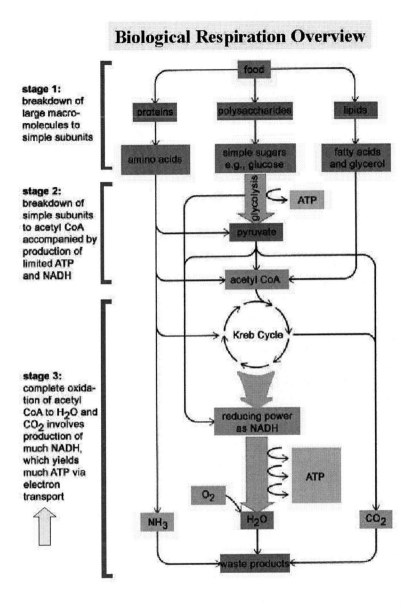

Biological Respiration Overview

stage 1:
breakdown of large macro-molecules to simple subunits

stage 2:
breakdown of simple subunits to acetyl CoA accompanied by production of limited ATP and NADH

stage 3:
complete oxidation of acetyl CoA to H_2O and CO_2 involves production of much NADH, which yields much ATP via electron transport

food

proteins — polysaccharides — lipids

amino acids — simple sugars e.g., glucose — fatty acids and glycerol

glycolysis → ATP

pyruvate

acetyl CoA

Kreb Cycle

reducing power as NADH

O_2

ATP

NH_3 — H_2O — CO_2

waste products

This is your body! As food comes in the top, chemical processing breaks down the energy packets into subunits and then into acetyl CoA with the production of the type of energy the body needs for its mitochondria, ATP. Note the **Krebs Cycle** is in the middle of the diagram which is more fully explained on the next page.

Krebs Cycle

Aerobic Respiration

The pyruvate produced in glycolysis undergoes further breakdown through a process called aerobic respiration in most organisms. This process requires oxygen and yields much more energy than glycolysis. Aerobic respiration is divided into two processes: the **Krebs Cycle**, and the **Electron Transport Chain**, which produces ATP through chemiosmotic phosphorylation. The energy conversion is as follows:

$$C_6H_{12}O_6 + 6O_2 \rightarrow 6CO_2 + 6H_2O + energy\ (ATP)$$

Krebs Cycle[177]

The pyruvate molecules produced during glycolysis contain a lot of energy in the bonds between their molecules. In order to use that energy, the cell must convert it into the form of ATP. To do so, pyruvate molecules are processed through the Kreb Cycle, also known as the citric acid cycle.

1. Prior to entering the Krebs Cycle, pyruvate must be converted into acetyl CoA (pronounced: acetyl coenzyme A). This is achieved by removing a CO2 molecule from pyruvate and then removing an electron to reduce an NAD+ into NADH. An enzyme called coenzyme A is combined with the remaining acetyl to make acetyl CoA which is then fed into the Krebs Cycle. The steps in the Krebs Cycle are summarized below:
2. Citrate is formed when the acetyl group from acetyl CoA combines with oxaloacetate from the previous Krebs cycle.
3. Citrate is converted into its isomer isocitrate.
4. Isocitrate is oxidized to form the 5-carbon α-ketoglutarate. This step releases one molecule of CO2 and reduces NAD+ to NADH2+.

---

5. The α-ketoglutarate is oxidized to succinyl CoA, yielding CO_2 and NADH2+.

6. Succinyl CoA releases coenzyme A and phosphorylates ADP into ATP.

7. Succinate is oxidized to fumarate, converting FAD to FADH2.

8. Fumarate is hydrolized to form malate.

9. Malate is oxidized to oxaloacetate, reducing NAD+ to NADH2+.

We are now back at the beginning of the Krebs Cycle. Because glycolysis produces two pyruvate molecules from one glucose, each glucose is processed through the Krebs Cycle twice. For each molecule of glucose, six NADH2+, two FADH2, and two ATP.

Electron Transport Chain

What happens to the NADH2+ and FADH2 produced during the Krebs cycle? The molecules have been reduced, receiving high energy electrons from the pyruvic acid molecules that were dismantled in the Krebs Cycle. Therefore, they represent energy available to do work. These carrier molecules transport the high energy electrons and their accompanying hydrogen protons from the Krebs Cycle to the electron transport chain in the inner mitochondrial membrane.

In a number of steps utilizing enzymes on the membrane, NADH2+ is oxidized to NAD+, and FADH2 to FAD. The *high energy electrons* are transferred to ubiquinone (Q) and cytochrome c molecules, the electron carriers within the membrane. *The electrons are then passed from molecule to molecule in the inner membrane of the mitochondron, losing some of their energy at each step.* The final transfer involves the combining of electrons and H2 atoms with oxygen to form water. The molecules that take part in the transport of these electrons are referred to as the "electron transport chain."

The process can be summarized as follows: *the electrons that are delivered to the electron transport system provide energy* to "pump" hydrogen protons across the inner mitochondrial membrane to the outer compartment. This high concentration of hydrogen protons produces a free energy potential that can do work. That is, the hydrogen protons tend to move down the concentration gradient from the outer compartment to the inner compartment. However, the only path that the protons have is through enzyme complexes within the inner membrane. The protons therefore pass through the channel lined with enzymes. The free energy of the hydrogen protons is used to form ATP by phosphorylation, bonding phosphate to ADP in an enzymatically-mediated reaction. Since an electrochemical osmotic gradient supplies the energy, the entire process is referred to as chemiosmotic phosphorylation.

Once the *electrons* (originally from the Krebs Cycle) have yielded

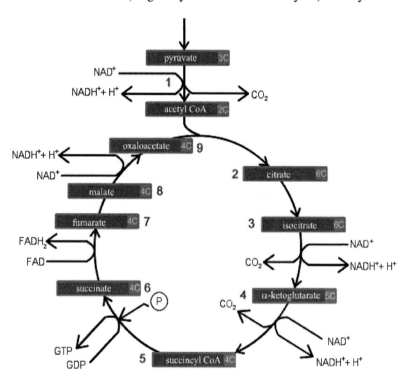

their energy, they combine with oxygen to form water. If the oxygen supply is cut off, the electrons and hydrogen protons cease to flow through the electron transport system. If this happens, the proton concentration gradient will not be sufficient to power the synthesis of ATP. The Krebs cycle may then revert to a fermentation cycle, powered by CO_2 instead, which encourages cancerous tissue formation.

100

Cell Membrane Electrical Strength and Electroporation

Dr. Panos Pappas
http://www.papimi.gr/theory.htm

The conclusion that the eukaryotic cell membrane may allow instantly and selectively the passage of an electrical charge on a particular ion is not fully understood, but the permanent dielectric strength of a eukaryotic cell membrane or its potential to insulate electricity is much higher than atmospheric air. Besides, the thickness of the cell membrane is extremely small in the range of some 10 Angstroms. This signifies that the cell membrane can stand 0.1 volts over a really microscopic barrier. The strength of the electric field is defined in physics as volts divided by distance (V/m). The corresponding strength of the field that is stopped by the membrane is thus 0.1Volts/10 Angstroms = $0.1V/10x10^{-10}m$ = 10,000 kVolts/meter. This means a **cell membrane can stand over ten million volts over a distance of one meter** while an atmospheric molecule or atmospheric air can stand only one million volts at the same distance! Atmospheric air within one meter from one million volts gets ionized and breaks down while cells do not! This is an incredible dielectric strength for the cell membrane.

The common, however less pronounced, effects observed with the other devices producing less peak power are also electroporation in origin phenomenon. Electroporation is not a phenomenon that starts just at a threshold of 1,000 volts/cm, but extends to a lesser extent below this value. Probably, the first stages of electroporation take place at down to 10 volts/cm or less, however, at a relatively lower rate. Electroporation, which opens the pores, e.g. sodium-potassium channels, is not fully understood and explained. Considering the above findings, we may attempt an explanation of the universal phenomenon of electroporation, based on very general principles of physics and living matter.[178]

Ed. Note: We caution against Dr. Pappas' PAP IMI device however.

---

[178] *Journal of Cellular Biochemistry,* 51:426, April 1993, J.C.Weaver of Harvard-MIT Division of Health Science and Technology, "Electroporation: A General Phenomenon for Manipulating Cells and Tissues"

Signal Discovery?

Mark Wheeler, March 2004, *Smithsonian*
http://www.smithsonianmag.si.edu/smithsonian/issues04/mar04/phe
nomena.html

A Los Angeles scientist says living cells may make distinct sounds, which might someday help doctors "hear" diseases.

Kids, lawn mowers, planes, trains, automobiles—just about everything makes noise. And if two California scientists are right, so, too, do living cells. In recent experiments using the frontier science of nanotechnology, the researchers have found evidence that yeast cells give off one kind of squeal while mammalian cells may give off another. The research, though still preliminary, is potentially "revolutionary," as one scientist puts it, and a possible, admittedly far-off medical application, is already being pursued: someday, the thinking goes, listening to the sounds your cells make might tell a doctor, before symptoms occur, whether you're healthy or about to be ill.

The founder of the **study of cell sounds**, or "**sonocytology**," as he calls it, is Jim Gimzewski, a 52-year-old UCLA chemist who has contributed to an art museum's exhibit on molecular structure. The cell sounds idea came to him in 2001 after a medical researcher told him that when living heart cells are placed in a petri dish with appropriate nutrients, the cells will continue to pulsate. Gimzewski began wondering if all cells might beat, and if so, would such tiny vibrations produce a detectable sound. After all, he reasoned, sound is merely the result of a force pushing on molecules, creating a pressure wave that spreads and registers when it strikes the eardrum. He also reasoned that although a noise generated by a cell would not be audible, it might be detected by an especially sensitive instrument.

Gimzewski is well suited to tackle the question, being both an expert at instrumentation—he has built his own microscopes—and comfortably at home in the world of the infinitesimal. A leader in nanotechnology, or the science of manipulating individual atoms and molecules to build microscopic machines, Gimzewski previously worked at IBM's research laboratory in Zurich, Switzerland, where he and his colleagues built a spinning molecular propeller 1.5 nanometers, or 0.0000015 millimeters in diameter.

They also built the world's smallest abacus, which had, as beads, individual molecules with diameters less than a single nanometer. If nothing else, the feats, which garnered considerable acclaim, showed that nanotechnology's much-hyped promise had a basis in reality.

For his first foray into sonocytology, Gimzewski obtained yeast cells from biochemistry colleagues at UCLA. (He "got looks," he recalls, when he explained why he wanted the cells.) Working with graduate student Andrew Pelling, Gimzewski devised a way to test for cellular noise with a nanotechnology tool called an atomic force microscope (AFM). Usually, an AFM creates a visual image of a cell by passing its very tiny probe, itself so small its tip is microscopic, over the cell's surface, measuring every bump and hollow of its outer membrane. A computer converts the data into a picture. But the UCLA researchers held the AFM's tiny probe in a fixed position, resting it lightly on the surface of a cell membrane "like a record needle," says Pelling, to detect any sound-generating vibrations.

The pair found that the cell wall rises and falls three nanometers (about 15 carbon atoms stacked on top of each other) and vibrates an average of 1,000 times per second. The distance the cell wall moves determines the amplitude, or volume, of the sound wave, and the speed of the up-and-down movement is its frequency, or pitch. Though the volume of the yeast cell sound was far too low to be heard, Gimzewski says its frequency was theoretically within the range of human hearing. "So all we're doing is turning up the volume," he adds.

The frequency of the yeast cells the researchers tested has always been in the same high range, "about a C-sharp to D above middle C in terms of music," says Pelling. Sprinkling alcohol on a yeast cell to kill it raises the pitch, while dead cells give off a low, rumbling sound that Gimzewski says is probably the result of random atomic motions. The pair also found that yeast cells with genetic mutations make a slightly different sound than normal yeast cells; that insight has encouraged the hope that the technique might eventually be applied to diagnosing diseases such as cancer, which is believed to originate with changes in the genetic makeup of cells. The researchers have begun to test different kinds of mammalian cells, including bone cells, which have a lower pitch than yeast cells. The researchers don't know why.

Few scientists are aware of Gimzewski's and Pelling's sonocytology work, which has not been published in the scientific literature and scrutinized. (The researchers have submitted their findings to a peer-reviewed journal for publication.) Word of mouth has prompted skepticism as well as admiration. A scientist familiar with the research, Hermann Gaub, chair of applied physics at the Ludwig Maximilian University in Munich, Germany, says the sounds that Gimzewski believes are cellular vibrations may have other origins. "If the source of this vibration would be found inside the cell, this would be revolutionary, spectacular, and unbelievably important," Gaub says. "There are, however, many potential [sound] sources outside the cell that need to be excluded." Pelling agrees, and says that he and Gimzewski are doing tests to rule out the possibility that other molecules in the fluid bathing the cells, or even the tip of the microscope itself, are generating vibrations that their probe picks up.

Ratnesh Lal, a neuroscientist and biophysicist at the University of California at Santa Barbara who has studied the pulsations of heart cells kept alive in a dish, says that Gimzewski's nanotechnology expertise may be the key to establishing whether cells produce sound. "The ultimate hope is to use this in diagnostics and prevention," says Lal, adding: "If there's anybody in the world who can do it, he can."

Gimzewski acknowledges more work needs to be done. Meanwhile, the findings have caught the attention of his UCLA colleague Michael Teitell, a pathologist specializing in cancers of the lymphocyte, a type of white blood cell. He's subjecting human and mouse muscle cells and bone cells to drugs and chemicals to induce genetic and physical changes; Gimzewski will then try to "listen" to the altered cells and distinguish them by their sounds.

Teitell says the thought of detecting cancer at its earliest cellular stages is exciting, but whether the technology will work as a diagnostic tool remains to be seen (or heard). He doesn't want to oversell the idea: "It could turn out that all these signals will be such a mishmash that we won't be able to clearly identify one from the other."

Gimzewski hopes the work will have a practical application, but the mere possibility that he's discovered a new characteristic of cells, with all the intriguing questions that raises, is, he says, "already more than enough of a gift."

Rife Pictures and Apparatus

Royal Rife Technologies
http://www.rt66.com/~rifetech/

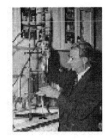

Rife at 60 years old

Rife Spectrum Analysis:
http://www.rifetechnologies.com/

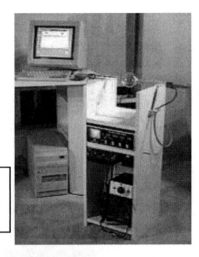

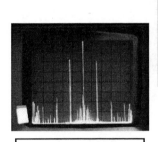

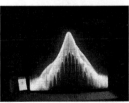

Rife EM Pulse
10 μs
(microseconds)

Rife Spectrum centered
At 27 MHz

Pulsed Technologies Rife Devices
http://www.pulsedtech.com/

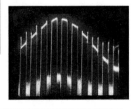

Rife spectrum at
5000 Hz

Chronology of R. Raymond Rife

- 1934 University of Southern California study - Pasadena City Hospital - 16 patients cured in 4 months with Rife Frequency Instrument

- 1938 *San Diego Eve. Tribune* **"devitalize disease organisms"**

- 1953 Rife's book, *History of the Development of Successful Treatment For Cancer, Virus, Bacteria and Fungi* published

- 1971 – Rife dies of Valium overdose

- 1972 *Cancer: A New Breakthrough* – published by Dr. Livingston-Wheeler

- 1968 – 1983 Dr. Livingston-Wheeler treats 10,000 patients with Rife Instrument and had an 80% success rate

- 1984 *The Conquest of Cancer* – second book by Dr. Livingston-Wheeler, USC

Websites: www.rife.org
www.keelynet.com/rife
www.kalamark.com
www.rifetechnologies.com

Patents: "Resonant Frequency Therapy Device"
1999, James E. Bare, #5,908,441

Curing Cancer with Ultra Radio Frequencies
by Georges Lakhovsky
Radio News (February 1925, pp. 1382-1283)
http://www.rexresearch.com/lakhov/lakhusps.htm

Since November 1923, I have published in various technical and radio publications, several papers in which I explained by theory that the instinct or special feeling, which permits birds to direct themselves in space, is only the results of the emission and reception of rays by living beings. While developing this theory, I explained how thoroughly I was convinced that science will discover, some day, not only the nature of microbes by the radiation which they produce, but also a method of killing disease bacilli within the human body by means of the proper radiations.

The researches I have made by means of special apparatus have shown such results, that I believe my theory is correct. This theory is that life is born from radiations, kept going by radiation and suppressed by any accident producing the destruction of the oscillator equilibrium, especially by the radiations of certain microbes, which suppress those of weaker cells.

Before going any further in our reasoning, it is necessary, in order to present the facts to the uninitiated reader, to imagine what oscillations really are. The motion of a pendulum will be used for this explanation. When a pendulum is displaced from the position of equilibrium, it moves back and forth producing what are known as ochrone oscillations, until the energy stored is entirely exhausted. By means of a motor, a spring, or an electromagnet, it is possible to keep the motion of the pendulum of constant amplitude, producing undamped oscillations. If, on the contrary, the source of power is removed, the oscillations die down and it is necessary not only to reapply the power sustaining the oscillations, but also to furnish additional energy to start the pendulum in motion. This oscillation of a pendulum reproduces exactly what happens in the cells of a living being.

Body Composition ~

Our organs are composed of cells formed of protoplasm containing mineral matters and acids such as iron, chloride, phosphorus, etc. It is by the combination of these elements that the cells detect outside waves and vibrate continuously at a very high frequency, probably higher than the period of x-rays or over all other vibrations known and measured today. The amplitude of cell oscillations must reach a certain value, in order that the organism be strong enough to repulse the destructive vibrations from certain microbes.

The astrophysicians are actually carrying out experiments of great interest on the existence of vibrations, which have been called penetration rays and of which the frequency is higher than that of x-rays and of the alpha, beta, and gamma rays of radium. Such rays, according to the theory, are produced by the earth itself and some others come from outside space. Some accurate measurements have proved the correctness of this theory. Therefore, it is quite permissible to believe that these penetration rays, or at least some of them, produce the vibratory motion of the living cells and consequently their life.

For instance, let us suppose a cell vibrates at a certain frequency and a microbe vibrates at a different frequency; the microbe begins to fight the cell, and sickness is started. If the cell cannot repel the stronger vibrations and if the amplitude of its own vibration decreases, the microbe gains and its vibrations succeed in decreasing and stopping those of the cells, bringing dangerous sickness or death. If, on the contrary, the living cell is started vibrating with the proper amplitude by inside or outside causes, the oscillatory attack is repulsed. Such is my theory. The problem is somewhat similar to the situation in which a rescuer finds himself when, coming to help a friend in a dangerous situation, finds himself fighting hand to hand against strong aggressors. The rescuer does not dare to fire his gun, fearing to harm his friend mixed up with the aggressors in the melee. Similarly, microbes and healthy cells are all exposed to electric or radioactive action, which could be used to destroy the unwanted rays and it is difficult to suppress them without harming or killing at the same time the cells which are to be treated. In fact, since Pasteur scientists have been constantly searching for means of destroying microbes. The great difficulty with all methods found was that in destroying, the bacillae cell was attacked too. The experience gained in cancer and tuberculosis treated with radium, or ultraviolet rays, shows how difficult is the work of the investigators.

A New Method ~

The remedy in my opinion, is not to kill the microbes in contact with the healthy cells, but to reinforce the oscillations of the cell either directly by reinforcing the radio activity of the blood or in producing on the cells a direct action by means of the proper rays. During January 1924, I began to build, according to this theory, and with the purpose of therapeutic applications, an apparatus, which I have called Radio-Cellulo-Oscillator, with the firm belief that the cells vibrating at extremely short wavelengths would find their own in the Hertzian waves, which have the properties of producing extremely short harmonics. The cells with very weak vibrations, when placed in the field of multiple vibrations, finds its own frequency and starts again to oscillate normally through the phenomenon of resonance. This type of vibration produced by radio waves which I propose to use, is harmless, unlike those of x-rays and radium. Their application, therefore, does not present any danger for the operator.

I exposed in front of my apparatus, during long periods, a certain number of microbes in culture, which developed themselves normally. I, myself, have never felt the effect of these ultra radio frequencies, although I remained for a great many days near the apparatus, during the treatment applied to the living cells. It is only when two living beings such as a cell and a microbe are in contact, that the rays produced by the Radio-Cellulo-Oscillator have any direct effect upon cellular structure.

The experiments which I carried out at the Salpetriere Hospital in Paris, in the service and with the collaboration of Prof. Gosset, were made with plants inoculated with cancer, and the results were described in a paper presented on July 26, 1924, before the Biological Society. The text of the paper follows:

"One knows that it is possible to produce by inoculation of bacterium tumefaciens in plants tumors similar to those of cancer in animals. One of us obtained experimentally by this method, a great number of tumors. These had various degrees of development. Some of them dry up partially, but do not die entirely until the entire plant or at least the limb bearing the tumor dies. Even removed by surgical methods, these tumors grew again on the sick limb.

The Radio-Cellulo-Oscillator ~

"We propose to describe in this paper, the action of electromagnetic waves of very high frequency obtained by means of the Radio-Cellulo-Oscillator of Georges Lakhvosky. This apparatus produces wavelengths of the order of two meters and less, corresponding to 150 million cycles per second. A first plant was submitted to the effect of the radiation one month after being inoculated with cancer; at this time small tumors the size of a cherry stone were visible upon it. This plant was submitted to the rays twice, for three hours each time. During the following days, the tumors continued to grow rapidly in the same way as those on plants which had not been submitted to the effect of radiations. However, 16 days after the first treatment, the tumors began to shrink and dry up. A few days later the tumors were entirely dried up and could be very easily detached from the limb of the plant by merely touching them. The drying action of the radio frequency radiations is selective and affects only the sick part of the plant. Even the inside sick tissues were destroyed, although they were next to healthy cells in the center of the limb, showing that the radiations had not affected the healthy parts.

The Length of Treatment ~

Another plant was treated in the same way, except that it was exposed 11 times, for three hours each time, to the radiations of the oscillator. Sixteen days after the first exposure the tumors, which were rather large as shown in one of the photographs, began to shrink and dry up and were easily detached form the limb exactly as in the first case. Again in this case, the healthy parts of the plant were not affected in the least. A third plant exposed to the radiations for 9 hours, that is, three treatments of three hours each, was cured in the same manner as the two others. Sixteen plants also inoculated with cancer, were left without treatment. They have tumors in full activity, several of which are very large. These experiments show conclusively that plants inoculated with cancer can be treated and cured by means of the ultra radio frequency vibrations, whereas surgical treatment fails.

"In conclusion I wish to call the attention of the reader to the fact that I have obtained very conclusive results not only with a wavelength of two meters, but with longer and shorter wavelengths. The main thing is to produce the greatest number of harmonics possible."

Such are the results of my researches with plants. At the present time, similar experiments are being carried out with animals and it seems that the effect on cancerous animals is the same as on cancerous plants.

I am highly pleased to present my theory and the results of my work in a scientific review of the United States, this great country, which has always been in the lead in this fight against this terrible sickness, cancer, and whose sympathy and help I would greatly appreciate.

Suggested References   (added by author for completeness)

Georges Lakhovsky, *The Secret of Life,* True Health Publishing Co., Rustington, Sussex U.K., third edition, 1963.

Grotz, T., B. Hillstead, "Frequency Analysis of the Lakhovsky Multiple Wave Oscillator from 20 Hz to 20 GHz" *Proceedings of the U.S. Psychotronics Association Annual Convention,* Portland, OR, July 1983 (The following three frequency spectra are sampled from the Toby Grotz article, also posted online.)

111

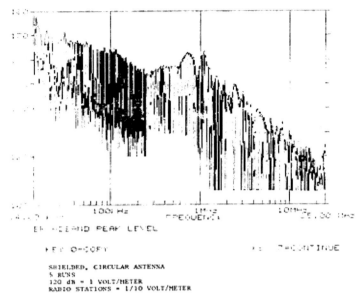

1) MWO Spectrum of 10 kHz to 25 MHz

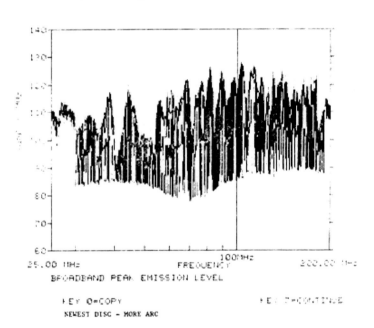

2) MWO Spectrum of 25 MHz to 200 MHz

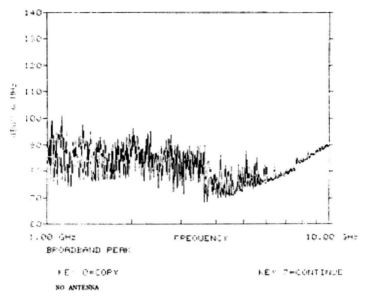

3) MWO Spectrum of 1 GHz to 10 GHz

<u>Author's Footnote:</u> As noted previously, the "**Lakhovsky Philosophy**" advocates the **bathing of the human body with a broadband of frequencies,** letting the body absorb what it needs. As seen above, the three ranges of frequency spectra, the kilohertz, megahertz, and gigahertz frequencies are included in a Tesla coil device, such as the Lakhovsky Premier 2000. This broadband bath may even include visible light pulses from the spark discharges, ultraviolet frequencies from the sparkgap and perhaps X-rays from tungsten electrodes in the sparkgap. The body can then absorb the frequencies that it needs and with the voltage boost to the TMP, the immune system can kick into gear with all of the tools it needs to do its complicated and integrated defensive work. In most cases, treatment with Tesla coil devices is a short term 5-15 minute exposure so as the cell phone study cited earlier in this book proved, the immune system is boosted. Along the same lines, a study has found that even exposure to safe levels of X-rays (4 millisieverts/year) doubles the level of glutathione, an antioxidant that protects cells, as reported in the *European Heart Journal* (10.1093) though peroxide free radicals were also increased. Cardiologist Tommaso Gori thinks it "makes you stronger."

113

Toroidal Coils and the Electromagnetic Vector Potential

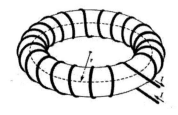

"Physics should be purged of such rubbish as the scalar (φ) and vector (A) potentials; only the fields E and B are physical," said 19th century physicist Heaviside, who was later proved wrong with the advent of quantum mechanics "which demands the vector potential."[179] Toroids for therapy may be studied more intently in the future because both E and B fields may be induced in the body at a distance without one being predominant, with an A potential <u>along the center</u> of the toroid (up or down in the above diagram). When A is pointed toward the body, the A potential can also offer the unusual property of inducing <u>circulating B fields</u> in tissue as well as <u>directed E fields</u>. B is the first derivative (curl) of A, where A diminishes as 1/r. Toroids (see #68 of Figure 9) can <u>change the momentum and phase of electrons nearby</u> by sending out a focused A potential through their center.

The force on a charged particle, such as ions in the body, is given by $F = qE$, where $E = -\partial A/\partial t - \text{grad } \varphi$. Therefore, a pulsed A potential will have the highest induced E field, when $\partial A/\partial t$ is large.

The "vector potential, although proven to be capable of interacting directly with electrons in a series of studies, is still ignored when designing electromagnetic devices and instruments of all kinds. Recent patent applications filed by Dr. Novak and his colleagues teach that the force of the vector potential, under certain electromagnetic field conditions (designated as concurrence-of-modes conditions), can directly affect electron states with consequences on a macro scale...a method for exciting the chemical bonds of molecules using an electromagnetic field. This method includes the steps of generating a plurality of electromagnetic oscillation modes." – Vector Energy Corporation http://www.venergycorp.com/tp_patent10040598.html

"The consequence of the Aharonov-Bohm effect is that the potentials, not the fields, act directly on charges."[180]

---

[179] Zee, A. *Quantum Field Theory in a Nutshell*, Princeton U., 2002, p. 217
[180] Imry, Y. et al. "Quantum Interference and the Aharonov-Bohm Effect" *Scientific American*, April, 1989, p. 56

Excerpt from Expert Declaration

DECLARATION OF THOMAS F. VALONE, No. C02-2240P – 4, Seattle-3209671.1 0053845-00002, January 19, 2004, STOEL RIVES LLP ATTORNEYS, 600 University Street, Suite 3600, Seattle, WA 98101-3197, Telephone (206) 624-0900

To summarize, the BELS unit[181] is simply a Tesla coil (including supporting circuit components such as magnetic core transformer, capacitor, spark gap, and air core resonant transformer) connected to light-emitting gas tubes.

The gas tubes are simply glass tubes (transparent or translucent) filled with specific gases which can be excited by high voltage exceeding 5000 volts to emit desired therapeutic frequencies of light.

The origin of the BELS circuit can be traced back to 1897 when Dr. Frederick Finch Strong performed experiments for therapeutic purposes with a tube of glass at the end of a Tesla coil, after the bare electrode proved to be painful to some patients. As he notes in his book documenting these experiments (*High-Frequency Currents,* Rebman Publishers, NY, 1908, p. 15), "It was but a step to substitute for the glass-covered metal electrode, a Geissler Vacuum Tube, in which the current passes through the body via the glass walls of the tube and the rarefied gas which it contains." Additionally, three conclusions can be drawn about this origin: 1) the Strong gas tube is specifically designed to be attached to the high voltage end of the Tesla coil for therapeutic purposes; 2) the discovery of this earliest prior art in the published literature has the same essential parts, arrangement, and purpose (means plus function); 3) while the Strong prior art presents only one gas tube at the high voltage end of a Tesla coil, the US Patent and Trademark Office (USPTO) routinely emphasizes that duplication of an invention for a multiplied effect is not held to be patentable.

Another historically famous use of the BELS circuit for decades is by R. Raymond Rife starting around the 1930's. As my book notes (*Bioelectromagnetic Healing: A Rationale for its Use*, Integrity Research Institute, DC, 2003, p. 11), Rife's circuit consisted of a "high voltage gas tube device." Specifically, in the 1930's this

---

[181] BELS stands for Bio-Electric Light Stimulator. - TV

usually necessitated the use of a Tesla coil to produce the high voltage. More importantly, Rife was the pioneering researcher who established the frequency relationships between high voltage gas tube light emissions and the microbe susceptibilities that provide the impetus for such BELS circuit use today.

The recent James Bare patent (#5,908,441) has supported his work by scientifically explaining the frequency and energy levels that are necessary in the high voltage gas tube excitation circuitry for the Rife technology to achieve its antiseptic properties. Rife subsequently published his book summarizing his life work entitled, *History of the Development of a Successful Treatment for Cancer, and Other Virus, Bacteria and Fungi,* Report No. Dev.-1042 Allied Industries, in 1953. It was published by Rife Virus Microscope Institute, San Diego, California....

.... As high voltage electrotherapy is re-discovered in the 21st century, it is ethically mandated to acknowledge the past century's contribution to the medical science which it represents. As a primary example, the BELS unit design has been established through the detailed historical citations to be a reproduction of Tesla technology already in the public domain.

Bone is Piezoelectric - actual electric signals recorded from weight-bearing force applied to a canine tibia   (Cochran, 1972)

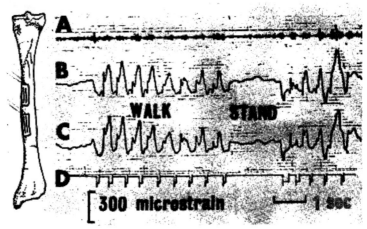

Fig. 3. Records from strain gages bonded to canine tibia: *A*, EMG; *B, C,* strains; *D,* foot contact. Since the physiologic electrical activity of bone is coupled with these mechanical strains, it seems logical that bone would be stimulated best by electrical pulses at similar frequencies.

Meditation Gives Brain a Charge, Study Finds

By Marc Kaufman, *Washington Post*, Jan 3, 2005, P. A05
http://www.washingtonpost.com/wp-dyn/articles/A43006-2005Jan2.html

Brain research is beginning to produce concrete evidence for something that **Buddhist practitioners of meditation** have maintained for centuries: Mental discipline and meditative practice can change the workings of the brain and allow people to achieve different levels of awareness.

Those transformed states have traditionally been understood in transcendent terms, as something outside the world of physical measurement and objective evaluation. But over the past few years, researchers at the University of Wisconsin working with Tibetan monks have been able to translate those mental experiences into the scientific language of **high-frequency gamma waves** and brain synchrony, or coordination. And they have pinpointed the left prefrontal cortex, an area just behind the left forehead, as the place where brain activity associated with meditation is especially intense.

"What we found is that the **longtime practitioners showed brain activation on a scale we have never seen before**," said Richard Davidson, a neuroscientist at the university's new $10 million W.M. Keck Laboratory for Functional Brain Imaging and Behavior. "Their mental practice is having an effect on the brain in the same way golf or tennis practice will enhance performance." It demonstrates, he said, that the brain is capable of being trained and physically modified in ways few people can imagine.

Scientists used to believe the opposite – that connections among brain nerve cells were fixed early in life and did not change in adulthood. But that assumption was disproved over the past decade with the help of advances in brain imaging and other techniques, and in its place, scientists have embraced the concept of ongoing brain development and "neuroplasticity."

Davidson says his newest results from the meditation study, published in the *Proceedings of the National Academy of Sciences* in November, take the concept of neuroplasticity a step further by showing that mental training through meditation (and presumably other disciplines) can itself change the inner workings and circuitry of the brain.

The new findings are the result of a long, if unlikely, collaboration between Davidson and Tibet's Dalai Lama, the world's best-known practitioner of Buddhism. The Dalai Lama first invited Davidson to his home in Dharamsala, India, in 1992 after learning about Davidson's innovative research into the neuroscience of emotions. The Tibetans have a centuries-old tradition of intensive meditation and, from the start, the Dalai Lama was interested in having Davidson scientifically explore the workings of his monks' meditating minds. Three years ago, the Dalai Lama spent two days visiting Davidson's lab.

The Dalai Lama ultimately dispatched eight of his most accomplished practitioners to Davidson's lab to have them hooked up for electroencephalograph (EEG) testing and brain scanning. The Buddhist practitioners in the experiment had undergone training in the Tibetan Nyingmapa and Kagyupa traditions of meditation for an estimated 10,000 to 50,000 hours, **over time periods of 15 to 40 years.** As a control, 10 student volunteers with no previous meditation experience were also tested after one week of training.

The monks and volunteers were fitted with a net of 256 electrical sensors and asked to meditate for short periods. Thinking and other mental activity are known to produce slight, but detectable, bursts of electrical activity as large groupings of neurons send messages to each other, and that's what the sensors picked up. Davidson was **especially interested in measuring gamma waves,** *some of the highest-frequency and most important electrical brain impulses.*

Both groups were asked to meditate, specifically on unconditional compassion. Buddhist teaching describes that state, which is at the heart of the Dalai Lama's teaching, as the "unrestricted readiness and availability to help living beings." The researchers chose that focus because it does not require concentrating on particular objects, memories or images, and cultivates instead a transformed state of being.

Davidson said that the results unambiguously showed that meditation activated the trained minds of the monks in significantly different ways from those of the volunteers. Most important, the electrodes picked up much greater activation of fast-moving and **unusually powerful gamma waves in the monks,** and found that the movement of the waves through the brain was far better organized and coordinated than in the students. The meditation novices showed only a slight increase in gamma wave activity while meditating, but some of the monks produced gamma wave activity more powerful than any previously reported in a healthy person, Davidson said.

The monks who had spent the most years meditating had the highest levels of gamma waves, he added. This "dose response" – where higher levels of a drug or activity have greater effect than lower levels – is what researchers look for to assess cause and effect.[182]

In previous studies, mental activities such as focus, memory, learning and consciousness were associated with the kind of enhanced neural coordination found in the monks. The intense gamma waves found in the monks have also been associated with knitting together disparate brain circuits, and so are connected to higher mental activity and heightened awareness, as well.

Davidson's research is consistent with his earlier work that pinpointed the left prefrontal cortex as a brain region associated with happiness and positive thoughts and emotions. Using functional magnetic resonance imagining (fMRI) on the meditating monks, Davidson found that their brain activity – as measured by the EEG – was especially high in this area.

Davidson concludes from the research that meditation not only changes the workings of the brain in the short term, but also quite possibly produces permanent changes. That finding, he said, is based on the fact that **the monks had considerably more gamma wave activity than the control group** even before they started meditating. A researcher at the University of Massachusetts, Jon Kabat-Zinn, came to a similar conclusion several years ago.

Researchers at Harvard and Princeton universities are now testing some of the same monks on different aspects of their

---

[182] For centuries, yoga practitioners have spoken about the "higher vibration levels" achievable through meditation. Science has finally caught up by proving that the highest electromagnetic vibration (frequency) level brain activity – gamma waves – increases in intensity the more deeply one meditates. (Gamma brain waves are in the range 20 – 80 Hz.) Furthermore, the author has witnessed high voltage bioelectromagnetics (Tesla coil, Lakhovsky MWO, and even a plasma globe) also triggering dramatic higher states of consciousness in those who meditate. - TV

meditation practice: **their ability to visualize images and control their thinking**. Davidson is also planning further research.

"What we found is that the trained mind, or brain, is physically different from the untrained one," he said. In time, "we'll be able to better understand the potential importance of this kind of mental training and increase the likelihood that it will be taken seriously."

More Information

"Introduction to Modern Meditation, Part II" *Explore*, Vol. 12, No. 1, 2003 by Thomas Valone (article summary) http://www.explorepub.com/articles/summaries/12_1_valone.html . Complete articles, Parts I & II, are reprinted in "Holistic Physics and Consciousness & Introduction to Meditation," IRI #401

Modern Meditation, Science and Shortcuts by Thomas Valone. Integrity Research Institute publishers, 103 pages, 2008. http://www.integrityresearchinstitute.org/Bioenergetics.html and Amazon.com

Why Electricity Can Heal the Body

"Electricity and rays are finer in nature than solids or liquids, and therefore a more subtle force for healing."

Paramahansa Yogananda, circa 1940
author of *Autobiography of a Yogi,*
Self-Realization, Winter, 2003 issue

Handheld PREMIER Junior

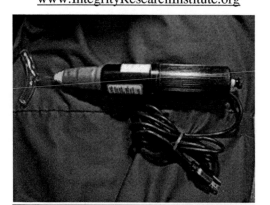

Model 100 with noble gas Y-tube

This product, designed by the author, evolved from the desire to provide a low-cost (few hundred dollar) alternative to the full-size Tesla coil and noble gas tube PEMF devices on the market today, as well as providing direct contact with the skin. It is a modern version of the Violet Ray and well insulated for daily use. PREMIER stands for Photon Rejuvenation Energizing Machine & Immunizing Electrification Radiator. One can use the **PREMIER Jr.** to boost TMP and receive electrons which preliminary studies show will directly fight free radicals. Invigorating and disinfecting, many people use it everyday to increase their resistance and relieve pain.[183]

PREMIER Jr. Models all come with Carrying Cases, 30-Day Return
Model 100 – Y-tube with high voltage coil and foam case
Model 200 – Mushroom tube with high voltage coil and foam case
Model 300 – Deluxe model with Y and mushroom tubes, high voltage coil and locking, instrument foam case
Model 500 – Professional model with Y-tube, two mushroom tubes (large and small), comb tube and locking, foam case
Model 2000—Lakhovsky antenna on a 100kV Tesla coil
 - One Year parts and labor Warranty, except glass tube breakage -
Integrity Research Institute, 5020 Sunnyside Ave, Suite 209, Beltsville MD 20705,   301-220-0440, **800-802-5243**
www.BioEnergyDevice.org   **IRI@starpower.net**

---

[183] This statement has not been approved by the FDA. The product is not intended to prevent, cure, treat, or diagnose disease.

PREMIER Jr. Product Line
www.IntegrityResearchInstitute.org

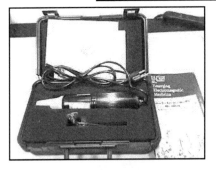

Model 200
With mushroom (round, flat end) gas tube and case

Model 300
with two tubes and 10"x 12" instrument case

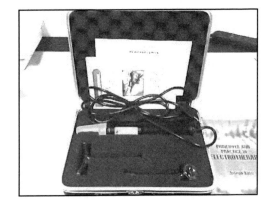

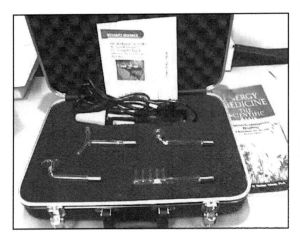

Model 500
with four tubes and 13"x 19" case

NovaLite 3000 - TeslaStar
www.NovaLite.com

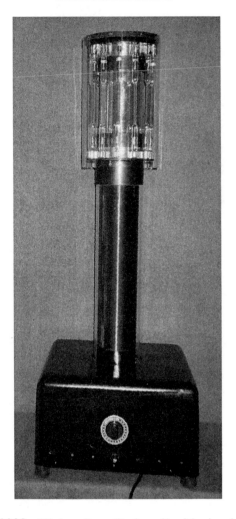

Novalite 3000 - High voltage Tesla coil with circular crown,
assorted noble gas tubes and timer, designed to stimulate and
balance body energy. Optional star crown configuration available
upon request (**TeslaStar**).
novalite@novalite3000.com
Novalite Research, Harvard Square, Cambridge, MA 02238
800-646-3622

Lakhovsky Multi-Wave Oscillator
PREMIER 2000
www.BioEnergyDevice.org

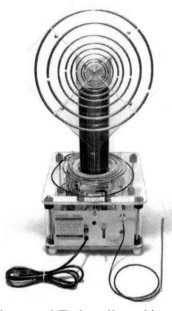

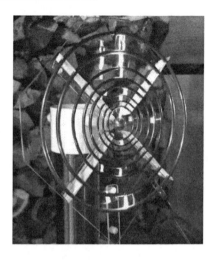

Perhaps the most durable Lakhovsky MWO on the market today. IRI has contracted with a manufacturer to offer this improved Tesla coil machine we call the **PREMIER 2000** with a wonderfully functional Lakhovsky antenna that radiates discrete frequencies in the RF band. This is a Tesla coil with the Lakhovsky antennas, antenna stand, cables and ground wire. Base enclosure and coil vinyl closure is optionally available for domestic use.

"I personally enjoy sitting in the multi-wave oscillator field because of the feeling of well-being it gives me." - William Bauer, MD

Integrity Research Institute
5020 Sunnyside Ave., Suite 209
Beltsville MD 20705
301-220-0440 800-295-7674
www.BioEnergyDevice.org

LBG
www.lightbeamgenerator.com
ELF Labs Tech 618-948-2393

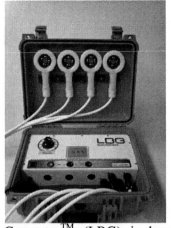

The Light Beam Generator^{TM} (LBG) is housed in a portable carrying case and uses a high voltage, high frequency output, powered by 14.5 volts DC with micro-current output. The LBG is a valuable tool for helping to restore proper functioning of the body's immune system defense. The LBG has enhanced manual massage efforts by over 90% and helped provide immediate relief from swollen conditions related to blocked lymphatics.

Jeff Spencer Erchonia PL-5 Therapeutic Pulsed Laser
http://www.roanokechiro.com/Chiropractic%20Therapies.htm

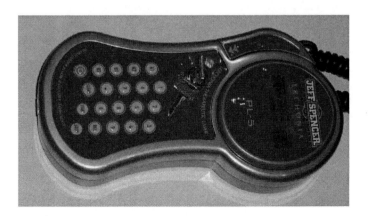

Electro-Acuscope Myopulse Therapy System
http://www.designmed.com/

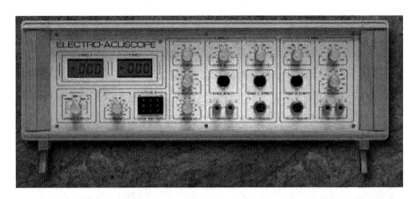

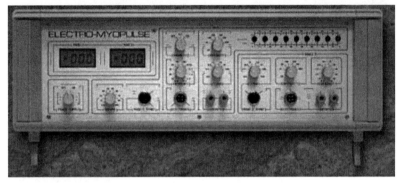

The Electro-Acuscope EAS-80L and Electro-Myopulse MYO-75L Therapy System is a highly sophisticated electronic medical instrument that has been applied to neuromuscular conditions commonly affecting equine athletes. The Acuscope uses electricity to treat pain by stimulating the nervous system without puncturing the skin. The Myopulse, a companion instrument to the Acuscope, gently stimulates muscles, tendons and ligaments, reducing spasm, inflammation and strengthening tissue damaged by traumatic injury. Treats: Bruising of muscle or fascia, Arthritis (acute chronic), Torn muscles, tendons, ligaments, Bursitis, Strain, Carpitis, Sprain, Laminitis (Founder), Rupture, Deep tissue infection, Hematomas, Cuts, Infections, Abrasions, Wounds, Abscesses, Incisions, Nerve paralysis, Necrosis, Muscle atrophy.
http://www.equiworld.net/uk/horsecare/alternativetherapies/electroacuscope/

Biomedical Design Instruments: info@designmed.com

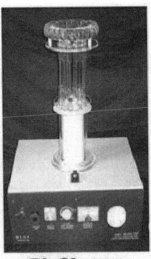

BioCharger
Advanced 1988

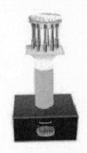
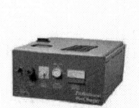

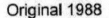
Original 1988   **BioCharger** Professional

BioCharger Corporation

This energy device is a high-voltage, high-frequency, resonant transformer (Tesla Coil) that transmits pulsed waves of electromagnetic energy wirelessly. The transmitted energy stimulates and invigorates the entire body on a cellular and subcellular level to optimize and improve health, wellness, and athletic performance. Results of an AIDS study are also online.

www.biocharger.com

Advanced Biotechnologies LLC **508-694-7824**

Medicinal Electromagnetic Fields

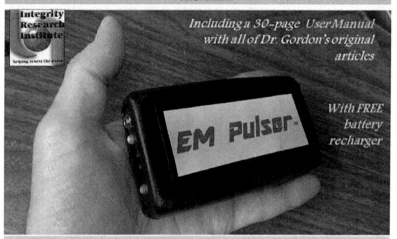

EM Pulser – New and Improved Version of Dr. Gordon's

Including a 30-page User Manual with all of Dr. Gordon's original articles

With FREE battery recharger

Rechargeable Internal Battery, More Powerful Pulse, Faster Pulse Rate, Bigger Coil, but still with the SAME Nanosecond Risetime!

View the PDF of the EM Pulser History and Operation online for a detailed explanation in slideshow format originally presented by Dr. Gordon and updated by Dr. Valone. EMpulse technology has always been safe and has never had a reported side effect. The new **EM Pulser** weighs five ounces in a 1" x 3" x 5" case and can be used at home, in the pocket, attached to clothing with Velcro® and is battery powered, as well as rechargeable (free charger included along with TWO rechargeable batteries). The EM Pulser is affordable a technology vastly superior to any other frequency devices and sells at a very competitive price. EM Pulser low frequency magnetic fields passes completely through your body to heal deep injury and relieve pain. Designed to activate the restorative and healing heat shock protein (HSP 70) within ten (10) minutes, with the famous "nanosecond rise time" pulses.

Integrity Research Institute
www.BioEnergyDevice.org
800-295-7674   301-220-0440

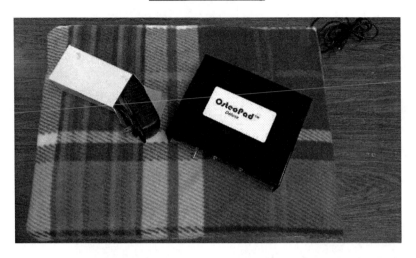

Inspired by the work of Drs. Bassett, Pilla, and Becker, IRI produced an affordable model for magnetic PEMF that also fulfills the dream of Glen Gordon M.D. for a <u>bone strengthening</u>, joint cartilage synthesis, and arthritis relief pad, that is also capable of **reversing osteoporosis** and osteopenia. As all four doctors discovered independently, pulsed magnetic fields dramatically open cellular calcium channels electrically. However, Dr. Gordon discovered that nanosecond rise time pulses are the most effective in creating a biological response in a short time as well as stimulating HSP 70. This product was developed with a pair of flat pancake coils, creating a toroidal magnetic field for better penetration while sleeping, along with a soft, flexible, vinyl sleeve covered with a flannel zipper case 15"x20". **OsteoPad Deluxe**, the most popular model with two pads, is also available for larger coverage, 30-day money back guarantee and one year warranty.

Integrity Research Institute
800-295-7674   301-220-0440
www.OsteoPad.org

Recommended Reading

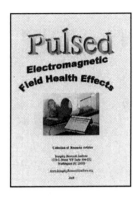

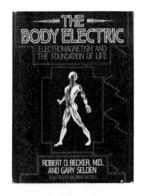

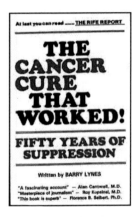

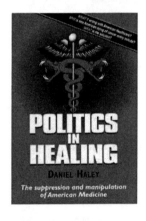

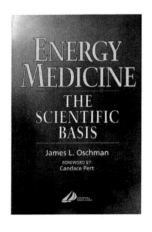

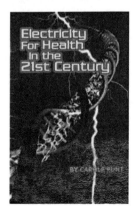

Integrity Research Institute Related Reports

Integrity Research Institute (IRI) is a non-profit corporation offering the following related reports. This book is published as part of the Bioenergetics Program. (Note, however, only the reports below are available through IRI, not the books recommended on the previous page.)

Pulsed Electromagnetic Field Health Effects – Resource guide report containing all of the latest scientific articles, data and abstracts related to PEMF research, including tissue trauma, pain treatment, bone strengthening, etc.
#418 / $15 / 60 pages

Bibliography of Bioelectromagnetism (BEM) – Two databases annotated with 600 references of titles and citations. Topics include how EMFs affect organs, nerves, behavior, histamine, calcium, and EEG.
#302 / $7 / 44 pages

Use of Electricity on the Face and Scalp by Emily Lloyd – Originally published in 1924, this reproduction contains complete protocols and directions for use of high voltage electrotherapy devices.
#419 / $20 / 120 pages

Medical Electricity CD by Sinclair Toussey, MD – Amazing four chapters, 1916 textbook on high voltage therapy and phototherapy with detailed photos and diagrams as well as patient responses. Adobe PDF format.
#416 / $15 / 250 pages

Energetic Processes: Interaction Between Matter, Energy and Consciousness, **Vol. I and II** by P. Moscow et al. – Two Anthologies with 20 papers on subjects such as hearing electrotherapy, energy machines, radionics, politics of electrical medicine, scalars, remote viewing, and alternative cancer therapy by PhD authors.
#413 / $25 / 480 pages and #415 / $25 / 400 pages

Visit www.IntegrityResearchInstitute.org or call 301-220-0440 (800-295-7674) for complete product catalog. Email: IRI@erols.com
----

NOTE: You are invited to email IRI@erols.com or mail a request for a **"FREE BEM's CD"** in the subject with your postal mailing address. The computer data CD (for Windows) includes a narrated BEM slide show, a NASA Study on PEMFs; "Biofields and Bioinformation" by Dr. Glen Rein; "History of Electromedicine" and much more.

IRI Rewards Page

FREE BONUS: A companion "Free BEMS CD" is available for free to those who have purchased this Book or eBook. It includes, among many other items, a NARRATED SLIDE SHOW in PowerPoint with audio dictated by the author. Email with mailing address to IRI@erols.com

Please send me a FREE IRI catalog-newsletter:

Name_____

Address_____

City_____ State_____ Postal Code_____

Country_____

Email_____

Where did you purchase this book?_____

Fax this form to 301-513-5728 or **Mail** to: Integrity Research Institute, 5020 Sunnyside Avenue, Suite 209, Beltsville MD 20705